THE CANDIDA CURE

Yeast, Fungus & Your Health

The 90-Day Program to
Beat Candida &
Restore Vibrant Health

~~~~~~~~~~~~~

Ann Boroch, CNC

Foreword by David Perlm
Author of *Grain B*

Quintessential Healing Pu   .C.
LOS ANGELES

ISBN: 978-0-9773446-1-1 (paperback)
ISBN: 978-0-9773446-3-5 (ebook)

15 14 13 12 11 10 9

Library of Congress Control Number: 2013936929

Published by Quintessential Healing Publishing, Inc.
Website: www.annboroch.com
Phone: 818.763.8282

For foreign and translation rights, contact Nigel J. Yorwerth
Email: nigel@publishingcoaches.com

Cover design: Geyrhalter Design
Website: www.geyrhalter.com

Interior design and production: Robert S. Tinnon Design

To the late Dr. William G. Crook:

As promised,

I carry on your mission

to help heal millions.

CONTENTS

FOREWORD

*At every crossway on the road that leads to the future,
each progressive spirit is opposed by a thousand men
appointed to guard the past.*

MAURICE MAETERLINCK
Belgian Nobel Laureate

Despite *Candida albicans'* thirty-year history as a well-defined and well-described clinical entity, the concept that a diverse range of seemingly disparate symptoms could be attributed to systemic overgrowth of this yeast species remains foreign to most medical practitioners. The unfortunate consequence of this naiveté is that countless sufferers of this malady, mostly women, know nothing about the medical and lifestyle interventions that can pave the way to their recovery.

The relative obscurity of this disease in mainstream medicine is not the only problem. Many of the time-honored practices of today's healthcare paradigm, including the excessive use of antibiotics and steroid medications—as well as the neglect of such simple practices as the use of probiotic beneficial bacteria—are actually setting the stage for the development of systemic candidiasis. As a result, those of us who deal with this health condition in the clinical setting are witnessing what now seems almost epidemic.

In the pages that follow, Ann Boroch provides the reader with a comprehensive understanding of this disease and its relevance to our health. Her firsthand personal experience coupled with extensive and exhaustive research has produced a text that will surely stand as a fundamental resource in the emerging story of candida as the hidden cause of many illnesses.

While *The Candida Cure* deftly weaves compelling text describing the magnitude of the problem, its causes and cures, the offering that shines most from its pages is summarized in one word—hope. For it is hope that is drained from the countless undiagnosed and inappropriately treated candida patients who stumble helplessly from doctor to doctor. And it is hope restored that is the highest merit of this book.

DAVID PERLMUTTER, MD, FACN, ABIHM
Naples, Florida
November 2008

PREFACE

Candida. Why write a book about a subject that most people don't know about? Because my personal journey of beating candida at age nineteen and then conquering multiple sclerosis (MS)—a disease related to candida— at thirty taught me how millions are suffering from this condition yet are in the dark as to why they feel so bad.

From as far back as I can remember, I was sick. I had many colds, flus, and sinus and ear infections. Throughout my life I was prescribed over a hundred courses of antibiotics for many different ailments. My diet until the age of eighteen consisted of processed foods filled with sugar, white flour, and trans fats. By the time I was thirteen, I had fifteen silver amalgam fillings from all the sugar I had eaten.

At nineteen, my body said no more and it collapsed from the Epstein-Barr virus, known as mononucleosis. Unfortunately, a few months of bed rest didn't turn my health around. After seeing eight different specialists, taking over thirty prescribed medications, and searching many months for answers on how to get well, I was still sick from head to toe.

Serendipitously, as I was hunting for answers in a bookstore one day, Dr. William Crook's book *The Yeast Connection* caught my eye. I scanned through the pages and went right to the questionnaire. I began to cry as I read the list of all of my symptoms—disoriented, poor memory, exhausted, upper respiratory infections, gastrointestinal complaints, weight loss, depression, etc. "Could this book be the answer?" I thought to myself. "Is yeast over-growth—candida—the root of what is wrong with me?"

I decided to take the plunge and follow Dr. Crook's program, which consisted of following a candida diet (no refined sugars, dairy, white flour, or alcohol) and taking an antifungal remedy called Nilstat. One long year later, I regained my health. In that one year, I discovered so much about how diet plays a critical role in getting rid of infection and inflammation, the root of disease.

Unfortunately, I did not know that I needed to maintain those healthy habits, and at twenty-four my life came to a grand halt when I was knocked flat with the diagnosis of multiple sclerosis. The doctor said, "Well, the great news is that you don't have cancer; the bad news is that you have multiple sclerosis. We have chemotherapy to experiment with." Terrified and shocked, I looked at my mother, who, offended by the doctor's insensitive manner, helped me hobble out of the office.

I then decided to find an alternative route to conquer the "incur-able disease." Finding my own answers was not easy—I had MS attacks daily for the first six to nine months, which kept me bed-ridden with fatigue, spasticity, tremors, numbness, tingling, and difficulty breathing, swallowing, and thinking. Two books that were instrumental in helping me build a framework to get well were Dr. Crook's book, *The Yeast Connection*, and Judy Graham's book, *Multiple Sclerosis*. To my dismay, I found very little information outside of these books about treating MS with alternative methods.

At a loss, I created my own self-help program and discovered that yeast and fungal toxins are the main culprit in all autoim-mune diseases. I went on a strict candida diet for four years, took an antifungal remedy, removed fifteen silver amalgam fill-ings, took nutritional supplements to heal the central nervous system, and worked through emotional and mental layers of fear-based patterns.

After four tumultuous years of dealing with MS symptoms and surviving a near-death experience and suicide attempt, I triumphed over MS at the age of thirty. In the last twenty-one years I have had no signs or symptoms of MS.

My healing triumph made it clear to me that my purpose was to help others heal. I decided to go back to school and became a naturopath and certified clinical hypnotherapist. I graduated from the International Society of Naturopathy as a naturopathic doctor and became a certified clinical hypnotherapist from the Holmes Hypnotherapy School. At thirty-two I opened my own practice in Los Angeles. A couple of years later I added to my credentials by becoming a certified iridologist from Bernard Jensen's International Iridology Practitioners Association and a certified nutritional consultant from the American Association of Nutritional Consultants.

At this writing, I have been in private practice for seventeen years. Running my practice and seeing thousands of clients has been an education in itself, yet my greatest insight into how to help others came from healing myself. Since then I have successfully treated all types of conditions, including allergies, autoimmune diseases, endocrine imbalances, gastrointestinal disorders, cancer, depression, anxiety, and more.

Having worked with so many health imbalances, I have come to the conclusion that candida overgrowth is pandemic and that treating it is the foundational place to start when working with any health condition or disease. I have found that clearing candida, along with other microbial infections (parasites, bacteria, viruses), removes the majority of infection and inflammation from the body and either eliminates symptoms altogether or gives me a clearer picture of the body system that is still out of balance.

The Candida Cure has come from my passion to get the work I do in my office out to the masses. In the first half of the book, you will learn what candida is and how most health imbalances start in the gastrointestinal tract. The second half of the book will teach you the difference between a poor and a good diet and give you all the information you need to create your own 90-day self-help treatment program and achieve a renewed level of health. You will find user-friendly charts, supplement protocols, a two-week sample menu plan, and delicious recipes that will help you to successfully eradicate candida overgrowth from your body.

Following my program will restore you to vibrant health and vitality within ninety days. The education and experience you will gain as you learn to listen and respond to the messages your body gives you when it is out of balance will empower you. And the wisdom of the changes you have made will prepare you to carry on with a lifestyle that promotes quality aging.

ACKNOWLEDGMENTS

I appreciate everyone who has helped me create this book. I would like to give special thanks to the following people: Janet Chaikin, for your copyediting and developmental editing, which have been impeccable—you are a godsend. Patricia Spadaro, for your overview and editing assistance. Nigel J. Yorwerth, for your invaluable guidance in helping shape, package, and market this book and for serving as my foreign rights agent. Bob Tinnon, for your interior design and production—you make it so easy. Aaron Silverman, Molly Maguire, Gabriel Wilmoth, and the SCB Distributors team, for distributing my books. Fabian Geyrhalter and the Geyrhalter Design team, for your creativity, which has captured and refined the essence of what my work has become. Armond Simonian, for your guidance and support in creating nutritional products that will help thousands. Dr. David Perlmutter, for being a great support and believer in the work that I do. Julie Jones-Ufkes, Andrea Berman, and Alison Moon, for your recipe contributions. And thank you to those who are very dear to me and always have my back—Jasmine Contor, Irene Zaragoza, and my mother!

PART ONE

THE HIDDEN CAUSE
OF MANY ILLNESSES

CHAPTER 1

THE CANDIDA EPIDEMIC

M any of the most common symptoms and illnesses that plague us today—from fatigue, bloating, and weight gain to prostatitis, brain fog, arthritis, allergies, depression, and multiple sclerosis—can be traced back to a surprising source. Yeast.

Yeast overgrowth, called candida, is pandemic today and affects millions. Conservatively speaking, one in three people suffers from yeast-related symptoms or conditions. While women immediately associate candida with vaginal yeast infections, men hear the word *fungus* and think it's the problem they're having with their toenails. But it's much more.

In addition to the conditions I've already named, candida is associated with persistent symptoms like ear and sinus problems, upper respiratory infections, PMS, fibroids, endometriosis, hypothyroidism, hypoglycemia, acne, and anxiety as well as more severe conditions such as autoimmune diseases, fibromyalgia, lupus, autism, mental illness, and even cancer.

How can yeast be such a significant health factor when so many don't even know about it? Simply because Western medicine continues to quietly ignore the connection between yeast overgrowth and the overuse of prescription drugs, especially antibiotics, and other common offenders, including diet and even the air we breathe.

WHAT IS CANDIDA?

Candida albicans is a harmless yeast, a type of fungus, that lives naturally in everyone's body: male, female, and child alike. In a healthy body, it lives symbiotically in a balanced environment in the gastrointestinal tract, on the mucous membranes, and on the skin. Unfortunately, this harmless yeast can overgrow and turn into an opportunistic pathogen.

As Dr. Michael Goldberg states: "Because it is a commensal organism [one that benefits from another organism without damaging or benefiting it] present in virtually all human beings from birth, it is ideally positioned to take immediate advantage of any weakness or debility in the host, and probably has few equals in the variety and severity of the infections for which it is responsible."[1]

Candida overgrowth and its by-products, mycotoxins, can attack any organ or system in your body. The attack is relentless, twenty-four hours a day, until treated. If not arrested, yeast, a single-celled organism, will change form—into a pathogenic fungus with roots that causes myriad symptoms. Throughout the book, I will be using the words *yeast* and *fungus* interchangeably.

This fungus burrows its roots into the intestinal lining and creates leaky gut—porous openings in the gut lining—which allows the fungus and its by-products to escape into the bloodstream. According to an article in the journal *Science*, "*Candida albicans* is the most common human systemic pathogen, causing both mucosal and systemic infections, particularly in immunocompromised people."[2] A systemic fungal infection is called candidiasis.

LIFESTYLE FACTORS THAT ENCOURAGE CANDIDA OVERGROWTH

The major causes of *Candida albicans* overgrowth are antibiotics, steroids (e.g., cortisone and prednisone), birth control pills, estrogen replacement therapy, poor diet, chemotherapy, radiation, heavy metals, alcohol overuse, recreational drugs, and stress. Other contributing factors include heavy metals in our silver amalgam fillings and the lead and cadmium in polluted air. All of the above directly or indirectly destroy the good bacteria in our gastrointestinal tract, allowing yeast to take over.

Yeast overgrowth thrives in the presence of diets high in refined sugars, refined carbohydrates, dairy products, alcohol, processed foods, and hormones secreted as a result of high stress levels. Acute and chronic stress elevates cortisol, a hormone produced by the adrenal glands (small glands that sit on top of each kidney). Excessive cortisol, in turn, raises blood sugar. The fungus doesn't care whether the increased sugar in your body is due to eating a candy bar or to having an episode of extreme stress; it will use the sugar as fuel to reproduce itself.

Once an imbalance occurs, yeast continues to multiply as it is fed by sugar in any form—alcohol, desserts, white flour, dairy products like milk and cheese, and elevated sugar levels caused by high stress. As years go by, mild to severe health conditions appear.

It is easy to see why the incidence of candidiasis is so high— the main contributing factors are various mainstream Western medicine protocols, rampant poor diet, and the stress overload so prevalent in our society today.

Western medicine may deny that yeast causes these myriad conditions, but the truth is that fungal toxins—the by-products produced by the yeast—disrupt cellular communication. Once that happens, inflammation and infection settle wherever we are genetically weak.

ANTIBIOTICS: CREATING A VICIOUS YEAST CYCLE

It takes only one dose of antibiotics in your lifetime to raise your yeast levels and create imbalances in your body. If you last took a course of antibiotics when you were ten years old, a poor diet and high stress levels will continue to feed the yeast over time until you begin to feel symptomatic.

North America, especially the United States and Canada, and pockets of Europe, have the highest numbers of people with candidiasis because Western medicine's standard protocol is to use antibiotic therapy for common infections.

A vicious cycle starts with the use of antibiotics (see Figure 1.1). For example, you have a cold or the flu and you visit your doctor, who prescribes antibiotics. The problem starts right there because colds and flu are viral infections, not bacterial ones, which is what antibiotics are designed for. Antibiotics are useless against colds and flu, yet many doctors prescribe them anyway. When you take the antibiotic it kills both good and bad bacteria in your gastrointestinal tract, as it cannot distinguish between them. Antibiotics do not affect *Candida albicans*, so without friendly bacteria like *Lactobacillus acidophilus* and *Bifidobacteria*, which keep the *Candida albicans* under control, the candida now multiplies.

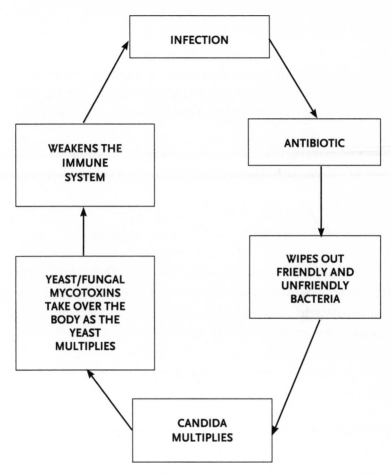

Source: Reprinted courtesy of William G. Crook,MD, *The Yeast Connection Handbook* (Jackson, TN: Professional Books, 2000). Used with permission.

FIGURE 1.1 The Vicious Cycle of Antibiotic Overuse

There is no question that antibiotics have saved thousands of lives, but we've pushed a good thing too far by overprescribing these medications. Overuse also creates "super germs" that are resistant to common antibiotics, so germs that could once be killed off have now become life threatening.

As I mentioned, it takes only one dose of antibiotics to raise your yeast levels. Think about how many times you've taken antibiotics—not to mention the antibiotics you ingest from consuming dairy and animal products. The majority of antibiotics manufactured today are given to cows and chickens because they are infested with infection due to their poor housing conditions. So unless you are eating antibiotic-free and hormone-free animal protein, you are ingesting these drugs and hormones when you eat these foods.

CANDIDA'S TOXIC BY-PRODUCTS

Once candida is in an overgrowth state, the body has to deal not only with the overgrowth but also with the toxic by-products, or mycotoxins, that *Candida albicans* puts out—"79 at latest count,"[3] according to C. Orian Truss, MD—all of which weaken your immune system and attack the body.

Mycotoxins are neurotoxins that destroy and decompose tissues and organs. They are so powerful that they upset the very communication of cell interactions, disrupt RNA and DNA synthesis, damage and destroy neurons, are carcinogenic, and cause ataxia (lack of coordination) and even convulsions. These pernicious yeast toxins confuse body systems, which accounts for the cross-wiring problems of the immune system whereby the body attacks itself, as in those with autoimmune diseases.

Candida toxins commonly get through the gut lining when it becomes leaky and enter the bloodstream, where the liver can detoxify them. However, if the liver's detoxification ability is impaired due to inadequate nutrition and toxic overload, these toxins will settle in other organs and tissues, such as the brain, nervous system, joints, skin, and so forth. Over time, chronic disease will occur.

TABLE 1.1. Damage from Acetaldehyde

Acetaldehyde Damages Brain Function

- Impaired memory
- Decreased ability to concentrate ("brain fog")
- Depression
- Slowed reflexes
- Lethargy and apathy
- Heightened irritability
- Decreased mental energy
- Increased anxiety and panic
- Decreased sensory acuity
- Increased tendency to alcohol and sugar
- Decreased sex drive
- Increased PMS and breast swelling/tenderness in women

Source: James A. South MA, *Vitamin Research Products Nutritional News*, July 1997.

One of the major toxins produced from *Candida albicans* is acetaldehyde (a by-product of alcohol metabolism), which the liver converts into a harmless substance. However, if there is an excess of acetaldehyde and the liver becomes oversaturated, it is released into the bloodstream, creating feelings of intoxication, brain fog, vertigo, and loss of equilibrium. Acetaldehyde alters the structure of red blood cells and compromises the transportation pathways whereby materials are delivered to feed the dendrites (nerve cell extensions), which causes the dendrites to atrophy and die off. In addition, acetaldehyde creates a deficiency of thiamine (vitamin B_1), a vitamin that is critical for brain and nerve function and essential for the production of acetylcholine, one of the brain's major neurotransmitters (see Table 1.1). This deficiency brings on emotional apathy, depression, fatigue, insomnia, confusion, and memory loss.

Acetaldehyde also depletes niacin (vitamin B3), which is key to helping the cells burn fat and sugar for energy. Niacin plays an important role in the production of serotonin, a neurotransmitter that affects mood and sleep, and in producing a coenzyme that breaks down alcohol. In addition, acetaldehyde reduces enzymes in the body that help to produce energy in all cells, including brain cells.

Gliotoxin, another mycotoxin, deactivates important enzymes that move toxins through the body and also causes DNA changes in the white blood cells, which suppresses the immune system. As your immune system continues to weaken from fungus and mycotoxins, more infections arise, and you end up at the doctor's office again—being prescribed more antibiotics and perpetuating the vicious cycle.

CANDIDA'S PREFERRED TARGETS

Candida albicans primarily targets the nerves and muscles, yet it can attack any tissue or organ, depending on your body's genetic predisposition (see Table 1.2). Mild symptoms of yeast overgrowth are fatigue, gas, bloating, heartburn, brain fog, weight gain, constipation, arthritic pain, sinus infections, high and low blood sugar, allergies, depression, and anxiety. More severe conditions can eventually develop, including autoimmune diseases and cancer.

To understand how candida penetrates through your system, think of your body as having two skins of protection that keep out foreign invaders. One is the outside skin and the other your

TABLE 1.2 Yeast/Fungal Overgrowth
(Conditions caused directly or indirectly by overgrowth)

Autoimmune Diseases
ALS (Lou Gehrig's Disease)
Chronic Fatigue Syndrome
Fibromyalgia
HIV/AIDS
Hodgkin's Disease
Leukemia
Lupus
Multiple Sclerosis
Muscular Dystrophy
Myasthenia Gravis
Rheumatoid Arthritis
Sarcoidosis
Scleroderma

Blood System
Chronic Infections
Iron Deficiency
Thrombocytopenic Purpura

Cancer

Cardiovascular
Endocarditis
Pericarditis
Mitral Valve Prolapse
Valve Problems

Digestive System
Anorexia Nervosa
Bloating/Gas
Carbohydrate/Sugar Cravings
Colitis
Constipation/Diarrhea
Crohn's Disease
Dysbiosis
Food Allergies
Gastritis
Heartburn
Intestinal Pain
Irritable Bowel Syndrome
Leaky Gut
Malabsorption/Maldigestion

Skin
Acne
Diaper Rash
Dry Skin and Itching
Eczema
Hives
Hair Loss
Leprosy
Liver Spots
Psoriasis

**Respiratory System/
Ears/Eyes/Mouth**
Asthma
Bronchitis
Dizziness
Earaches
Environmental Allergies/
    Chemical Sensitivities
Hay Fever
Oral Thrush
Sinusitis

Endocrine System
Adrenal/Thyroid Failure
Diabetes
Hormonal Imbalances
Hypoglycemia
Insomnia
Over/Underweight

Nervous System
Alcoholism
Anxiety
Attention Deficit Disorder
Autism
Brain Fog
Depression
Headaches
Hyperactivity
Hyperirritability
Learning Difficulties
Manic-Depressive Disorder
Memory Loss
Migraines
Schizophrenia
Suicidal Tendencies

Urinary/Reproductive
Cystitis
Endometriosis
Fibroids
Impotence
Loss of Libido
Menstrual Irregularities
PMS
Prostatitis
Sexually Transmitted Diseases
Urethritis
Yeast Vaginal Infections

Virus
Epstein-Barr Virus

inside skin, which starts in your nasal passages and runs all the way down to your rectum. This tissue is the same from top to bottom, and if it becomes inflamed or irritated, the membranes become more porous, allowing foreign invaders to enter the bloodstream. In the journal *Infection and Immunity*, Michael J. Kennedy and Paul A. Volz explain, "The passage of viable *Candida albicans* through the gastrointestinal (GI) mucosa into the bloodstream is believed to be an important mechanism leading to systemic candidosis."[4]

Cellular disruption occurs when *Candida albicans* and its mycotoxins have accumulated in the body. This disruption causes secondary body systems to deteriorate. Mycotoxins so severely debilitate the body that "victims could become easy prey for far more serious diseases such as acquired immune deficiency syndrome, multiple sclerosis, rheumatoid arthritis, myasthenia gravis, colitis, regional ileitis, schizophrenia, and possibly death from candida septicemia," say Kennedy and Volz.[5] Your genetic weaknesses usually determine which system or organs will be affected.

SETTING OFF A CASCADE OF IMBALANCES

Candida overgrowth creates a cascade of imbalances in the body. Three major areas worth noting are the proliferation of other microorganisms, imbalances in the hormonal system, and emotional disturbances, especially anxiety and depression.

Bacteria, Parasites, and Viruses

Unfortunately, once the body's internal environment is out of balance, not only does candida multiply but so do other microorganisms. Why? Because a poor diet and/or high stress levels elevate blood sugar in the body, which in turn feeds bacteria, parasites, and viruses. One of the most common viral infections, Epstein-Barr virus, also known as mononucleosis, cannot surface without the presence of yeast overgrowth. Therefore, when treating candida, I suggest using a broad-spectrum antimicrobial herbal remedy that addresses not only yeast and fungus but bacteria, parasites, and viruses as well.

Endocrine Imbalances

Candida overgrowth indirectly impacts the functioning of the endocrine system, which releases hormones that regulate the body's metabolic activity. The endocrine system consists of the hypothalamus, pituitary, thyroid, thymus, adrenals, pancreas, and ovaries or testes.

Problems related to these glands and organs include low blood sugar (hypoglycemia), diabetes, and obesity, all of which are increasing at alarming proportions in the United States. Hypothyroidism is rampant, especially among women. And the ailment most common across the board with males and females is adrenal exhaustion, where the adrenals output chronically high cortisol levels, resulting in fatigue, low immunity, anxiety, insomnia, and weight gain.

The primary aggravators of these conditions are a poor diet, consisting of refined carbohydrates and sugar, and unmanaged stress. The secondary aggravator is yeast overgrowth.

Over the years, I have had many clients say to me, "Why can't I lose weight? I'm eating healthy foods and exercising and can't drop a pound." The missing link is clearing the body of infection by getting rid of candida overgrowth, which eliminates

inflammation and allows the body systems to normalize. Eradicate candida and watch the inches and pounds drop as your
endocrine system comes back into balance.

Emotional and Mental Imbalances

Depression and anxiety are widespread and can, in part, be
related to chronic yeast overgrowth in the tissues. The reason,
as described by J. P. Nolan in an article in the journal *Hepatology*, is the link between the gut and the brain: "An individual's
ability to protect against brain-active substances depends upon
the status of his or her intestinal flora, GI mucosal function
and hepatic (liver) detoxification ability."[6] This means that when
leaky gut is present and the liver is overstressed, the door is open
for toxins to reach the brain via the bloodstream.

Unfortunately, too many physicians assume that all mental
and emotional imbalances have psychological causes, such as
neuroses or psychoses, rather than brain-related causes, as Dr.
C. Orian Truss points out in *The Missing Diagnosis*:

> I would like to make a special plea that we speak of manifesta-
> tions of abnormal brain function not as "mental symptoms" but
> as "brain symptoms." Inherent in the term "mental symptom"
> is the connotation that somehow "the mind" is a separate entity
> from the brain, that "mental" symptoms are occurring (at least
> initially) in a brain that is functioning normally chemically and
> physiologically. We speak of kidney, liver, or intestinal symptoms
> when abnormal function manifests itself in these organs, but we
> use the term "mental symptoms" rather than "brain symptoms"
> when a similar problem occurs with brain physiology.[7]

Having anxiety and/or depression can be debilitating, and it's important to understand that the cause may not be purely psychological but also chemical. Mycotoxins from fungus need to be considered when tackling these conditions. When this is a contributing factor, clearing fungal overgrowth from the system will help clear your mind and bring your body chemistry back into balance.

WESTERN MEDICINE'S DENIAL

To this day, Western medicine does not recognize intestinal and systemic candidiasis as a health condition. Don't be surprised if you take this information to your doctor and he or she dismisses it or tells you that you are crazy. Often doctors only recognize and treat *Candida albicans* overgrowth in cases of oral thrush and vaginal infections or in conditions associated with HIV/AIDS.

With antibiotics, hormone replacement drugs, birth control pills, and steroid drugs accounting for millions of dollars in prescriptions written each year, doctors are going to be the last ones to acknowledge that the drugs they so freely prescribe are actually creating the problem and that intestinal candidiasis even exists. While there are some doctors who will treat intestinal and systemic candidiasis, they are few and far between.

DO I HAVE CANDIDA?

The following questionnaire will help you determine whether *Candida albicans* is contributing to your health problems, but it won't provide an automatic yes or no answer. Even if you score low on this test, indicating a lesser possibility of candida, I still recommend that you follow my 90-day program since the typical lifestyle habits of most people today make it almost certain that you have a mild to moderate case of yeast overgrowth. It's challenging to come up with exactly the right test, whether written or in the laboratory, to confirm candida overgrowth.

The questionnaire, developed by William G. Crook, MD, lists factors in your medical history that promote the growth of *Candida albicans* (Section A) as well as symptoms commonly found in individuals with yeast-connected illness (Sections B and C).

Candida Health Questionnaire

For each "yes" answer in Section A, circle the point score next to the question. Total your score, and record it at the end of the section. Then move on to Sections B and C and score as directed. At the end of the questionnaire, you will add your scores to get your grand total.

SECTION A: History   Point Score

1. Have you taken any tetracyclines (Sumycin, Panmycin, Vibramycin, Minocin, etc.) or other antibiotics for acne for one month (or longer)? (50)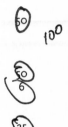

2. Have you at any time in your life taken other "broad spectrum" antibiotics for respiratory, urinary or other infections for two months or longer, or for shorter periods four or more times in a one-year span? (50)

3. Have you taken an antibiotic drug—even for one round? 6

4. Have you at any time in your life been bothered by persistent prostatitis, vaginitis, or other problems affecting your reproductive organs? (25)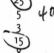

5. Have you been pregnant two or more times? 5
   One time? 3

6. Have you taken birth control pills for more than two years? (15)
   For six months to two years? 8

7. Have you taken prednisone, Decadron, or other cortisone-type drugs by mouth or inhalation for more than two weeks?* (15)
   For two weeks or less? 6

8. Does exposure to perfumes, insecticides, fabric shop odors, or other chemicals provoke moderate to severe symptoms? 20
   Mild symptoms? 5

9. Are your symptoms worse on damp, muggy days or in moldy places? (20)

10. Have you had athlete's foot, ringworm, "jock itch," or other chronic fungus infections of the skin or nails? (20)
    Have such infections been severe or persistent? (20)
    Mild to moderate? (10)

11. Do you crave sugar? (10)

12. Do you crave breads? 10

13. Do you crave alcoholic beverages? (10)

14. Does tobacco smoke really bother you? 10

Total Score, Section A   _____

*The use of nasal or bronchial sprays containing cortisone and/or other steroids promotes overgrowth in the respiratory tract.

Source: This questionnaire is adapted from William G. Crook, MD, *The Yeast Connection Handbook* (Jackson, TN: Professional Books, Inc, 2000). Used with permission.

SECTION B: Major Symptoms

For each symptom you experience, enter the appropriate number in the point score column:

> If a symptom is occasional or mild, score 3 points.
> If a symptom is frequent and/or moderately severe, score 6 points.
> If a symptom is severe and/or disabling, score 9 points.

Total the score and record it at the end of this section.

Point Score

1.	Fatigue or lethargy	3
2.	Feeling "drained"	3
3.	Poor memory	
4.	Feeling "spacey" or "unreal"	3
5.	Inability to make decisions	
6.	Numbness, burning, or tingling	6
7.	Insomnia	
8.	Muscle aches	
9.	Muscle weakness or paralysis	
10.	Pain and/or swelling in joints	
11.	Abdominal pain	
12.	Constipation	9
13.	Diarrhea	
14.	Bloating, belching, or intestinal gas	
15.	Troublesome vaginal burning, itching, or discharge	
16.	Prostatitis	
17.	Impotence	
18.	Loss of sexual desire or feeling	
19.	Endometriosis or infertility	
20.	Cramps and/or other menstrual irregularities	
21.	Premenstrual tension	
22.	Attacks of anxiety or crying	3
23.	Cold hands or feet and/or chilliness	
24.	Shaking or irritability when hungry	

27

Total Score, Section B _____

SECTION C: Other Symptoms*

For each symptom you experience, enter the appropriate number in the point score column:

> If a symptom is occasional or mild, score 3 points.
> If a symptom is frequent and/or moderately severe score, 6 points.
> If a symptom is severe and/or disabling score, 9 points.

Total the score and record it at the end of this section.

*Although the symptoms in this section occur commonly in patients with yeast-connected illness, they also occur commonly in patients who do *not* have candida.

Point Score

1. Drowsiness   2
2. Irritability or jitteriness   3
3. Lack of coordination
4. Inability to concentrate   6   12
5. Frequent mood swings
6. Headaches   3
7. Dizziness and/or loss of balance
8. Pressure above ears or feeling of head swelling
9. Tendency to bruise easily   9   24
10. Chronic rashes or itching
11. Psoriasis or recurrent hives
12. Indigestion or heartburn   6   36
13. Food sensitivities or intolerances   6
14. Mucus in stools
15. Rectal itching
16. Dry mouth or throat
17. Rash or blisters in mouth
18. Bad breath
19. Foot, hair, or body odor not relieved by washing
20. Nasal congestion or postnasal drip
21. Nasal itching
22. Sore throat
23. Laryngitis or loss of voice
24. Cough or recurrent bronchitis
25. Pain or tightness in chest   9   48
26. Wheezing or shortness of breath
27. Urinary frequency, urgency, or incontinence
28. Burning on urination
29. Erratic vision or spots in front of eyes
30. Burning or tearing of eyes   3
31. Recurrent infections or fluid in ears
32. Ear pain or deafness

Total Score, Section C   48
Total Score, Section B   27
Total Score, Section A   221
Grand Total Score (Add totals from sections A, B, and C)   296

The Grand Total Score will help you and your practitioner decide if your health problems are yeast-connected. Scores for women will run higher because seven items apply exclusively to women, while only two apply exclusively to men.

- Yeast-connected health problems are almost certainly present in women with scores over 180 and in men with scores over 140.

- Yeast-connected health problems are probably present in women with scores over 120 and in men with scores over 90.
- Yeast-connected health problems are possibly present in women with scores over 60 and in men with scores over 40.
- Scores of less than 60 for women and less than 40 for men indicate that yeast are less apt to cause health problems.

CHAPTER 2

THE DIGESTIVE SYSTEM AND THE ORIGIN OF DISEASE

One of the most overlooked systems of the body is the digestive system. An imbalance in this system—comprised of the mouth, salivary glands, stomach, pancreas, liver, gallbladder, and small and large intestines—is responsible for the onset of the majority of health conditions and chronic progressive diseases plaguing Americans (see Figure 2.1).

While there has been a lot of attention focused these days on the importance of a healthy immune system, few people realize that about 80 percent of the immune system's cells are produced in the digestive tract. For this reason, no matter what condition a client is experiencing, I always start them off with my foundational program of cleansing and rebalancing the digestive system. I'm still shocked to see some top medical specialists continue to ignore diet and infection (including candida) as the source of serious gastrointestinal conditions, including ulcerative colitis and Crohn's disease, even after their treatments consistently fail to help their patients, many of whom end up in my office.

As naturopath Mark Percival states in *Functional Dietetics:* "Destructive eating habits lead first to gastrointestinal dysfunction and then subsequently contribute to virtually every noninfectious disease known to us (and likely some of the infectious diseases as well)."[1]

Scientists tell us that there are ten times more bacterial cells living inside the gastrointestinal tract (GI tract), the stomach, and intestines than there are human cells in the entire body. The small and large intestines alone have a combined length of twenty to twenty-five feet, the width of a tennis court if you stretch them out. A balanced ecosystem in the GI tract has a ratio of 80 percent healthy microorganisms to 20 percent unhealthy ones. Inadequate diets based on foods that are depleted of nutrients and filled with chemicals and preservatives upset this ratio and can create maldigestion, malabsorption, intestinal dysbiosis (overgrowth of microbes such as fungi, parasites, bacteria, and viruses in the gut), and elimination problems. What's more, these problems are not isolated conditions that affect just the digestive system; they also affect other systems of the body, including the immune system.

MALDIGESTION:
THE CAUSE OF INDIGESTION

Maldigestion occurs when the body is unable to properly break down food. Reasons for this include lack of hydrochloric acid (HCl) in the stomach, inadequate chewing, poor food combining, excessive drinking of liquids with meals, pancreatic enzyme deficiencies, hiatal hernia, and stress. Chronic poor diet contributes to maldigestion.

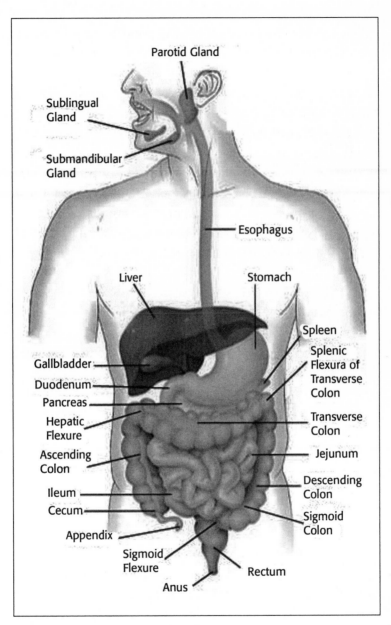

FIGURE 2.1 Anatomy of the Digestive System

When food goes undigested, the particles create toxic by-products that irritate the intestinal walls and cause increased permeability. The toxins can then cross the mucosal lining, where they enter the bloodstream (leaky gut syndrome). The blood sees these particles as foreign invaders and creates an antibody response by having the white blood cells come to the rescue to defend your body. However, this activity produces inflammation, allergic reactions, and food sensitivities. In addition, the undigested food particles produce fermentation, which fuels fungal overgrowth and the proliferation of bacteria and parasites. Symptoms of maldigestion include belching, bloating, gas, abdominal pain, and heartburn.

ENZYME DEFICIENCIES

Enzyme deficiencies are a major contributor to maldigestion. Enzymes are proteins that act as catalysts to ignite chemical reactions in the body. While the body does manufacture its own enzymes, it must also make use of those in food to have optimal health. Most enzymes are destroyed in foods that are processed, refined, or cooked at temperatures above 118 degrees. Raw or lightly steamed foods, on the other hand, are rich in enzymes.

When enzymes are lacking in the body, the pancreas, which secretes digestive enzymes, takes on a greater load. The pancreas also has the job of producing insulin, the hormone that maintains blood sugar levels. Therefore, diets loaded with refined carbohydrates, sugar, and cooked and processed foods overwork the pancreas and weaken its performance, making us more susceptible to yeast overgrowth and conditions like hypoglycemia and diabetes.

MALABSORPTION AND
THOSE UNEXPLAINED COMPLAINTS

Malabsorption occurs when the uptake of food from the intestines is impaired. Without proper absorption, you cannot nourish your cells, and they begin to degenerate. Nutrients are absorbed from food by villi (hairlike projections), but a poor diet and toxic overload in the body can strip the villi and inhibit their function, creating malabsorption.

The main causes of malabsorption are maldigestion and microbial overgrowth (bacteria, yeast, parasites, worms, and viruses). Common symptoms of malabsorption are fatigue, thinning hair, dry skin, depression, susceptibility to bruising, unexplainable weight loss, and constipation or diarrhea.

DYSBIOSIS AND UNWELCOME INHABITANTS

Intestinal dysbiosis is an imbalance of microorganisms (yeast, bacteria, parasites, and viruses), which upsets the digestive system and interferes with nutrient absorption. Dysbiosis is caused by poor diet; alcohol; recreational drugs; stress; maldigestion; elimination problems; the overuse of antibiotics; steroids such as cortisone, prednisone, and birth control pills; nonsteroidal anti-inflammatory drugs (NSAIDs); heavy metal toxins; and immunosuppressive drugs.

When unhealthy microorganisms take over the gut, your immune system is put under constant stress to defend your body from these infections. Intestinal dysbiosis is a contributing cause in rheumatoid arthritis, MS, vitamin B_{12} deficiency, chronic fatigue, cystic acne, the early stages of colon and breast cancers, eczema, food allergies and sensitivities, inflammatory bowel disease, irritable bowel syndrome, psoriasis, Sjögren's syndrome (a postmenopausal immunological disorder), and steatorrhea (excess fat in the stools). The most common form of intestinal dysbiosis is *Candida albicans* overgrowth.

LEAKY GUT SYNDROME

Maldigestion, malabsorption, and intestinal dysbiosis set the stage for leaky gut syndrome. As I've discussed, leaky gut is a condition in which the intestines' mucosal lining becomes irritated, inflamed, and more porous, allowing undigested food particles, microorganisms, and their by-products to pass through the lining into the bloodstream. Candida overgrowth, NSAIDs, poor diet, heavy metals, daily aspirin use, and gluten sensitivity to wheat, spelt, kamut, rye, barley, triticale, white flour, and oats (due to cross-contamination) all contribute to irritating the lining.

"Leaky gut triggers a state of continuous and prolonged stress in and on the immune system," says Dr. Jeffrey S. Bland.[2] Allergies are one of the first conditions to occur when someone has leaky gut. Other more serious conditions may follow.

The gut lining, as I explained in Chapter 1, acts as a protective mucosal barrier and is your first line of defense to prevent infection. When pathogens and foreign organisms come into contact with the mucosal barrier, immune cells inside the gut produce secretory immunoglobin A (SigA), an antibody that attacks them. However, chronic stress continually suppresses SigA production and thus allows pathogens to enter your bloodstream and eventually migrate to your brain and other tissues.

Over time, the presence of bacteria, yeast, parasites, and viruses traveling in the bloodstream means that the body is under siege. As these toxins circulate in the bloodstream, organs such as the liver, the lymph glands, the brain, the lungs, and the kidneys become overloaded. When cellular communication is disrupted, cross-wiring of the RNA and DNA and the replication of unhealthy cells result, leading to autoimmune diseases and cancer. Simply put, leaky gut causes chronic inflammation, which eventually translates to disease.

LEAKY GUT AND THE LIVER

The liver is an amazing organ. The largest in the body, it has more than five hundred functions. You can't live without your liver. It assists with metabolism, storing vitamins and minerals, and detoxifying toxic compounds.

Here's just a small piece of the picture. The portal vein delivers blood from the small intestine to the liver containing not only nutrients from digested food, but also toxins. The nutrients are carried through the circulatory system to feed every cell of your body. But what happens to the toxins?

One of the liver's many tasks is to recognize and neutralize these poisons, which come from substances such as heavy metals, pesticides, toxic foods, alcohol, cigarettes, synthetic chemicals, medications, and the by-products of stress hormones. Leaky gut makes the job of the liver more difficult by forcing it to break down undigested proteins as well as deal with the microbes and their by-products that have entered it through the blood. If the liver can't keep up with the overload of toxins, they will be stored in the liver or recirculated in the body. The combined effect is an interference with the liver's efficiency.

The liver produces and secretes bile, which is stored in the gallbladder until it is needed by the small intestine to assist with fat digestion. In addition to breaking down fats and its other important roles, bile has antibacterial properties that help protect the small intestine from harmful bacteria, yeast, and parasites. However, in a toxic body bile often becomes thick and sludgy, hampering its flow and function. One result is that yeast, viruses, and bacteria flourish, upsetting the ratio of good to bad bacteria.

The function of bile can be compromised by an excess of estrogen hormones, which reduces bile flow and elevates bile cholesterol levels. This poses a risk of gallstones and the recirculation of estrogens, increasing the risk of cancers of the breast, ovaries, uterus, and prostate.

An impaired liver can lead to problems in another important area. An article in the journal *Lancet* states: "When the gut becomes leaky, more toxic substances are delivered to the liver, and if the liver's functional ability to detoxify is impaired, more metabolically active substances are delivered through the bloodstream to other tissues, including the brain."[3]

Like the GI tract lining, the blood-brain barrier can become compromised. When this happens, toxins that escape the liver become stored in fatty tissues, such as the cells of the brain and the central nervous system, causing inflammation and oxidative stress. This accounts for the wide range of noninfectious diseases you see today, specifically MS, Parkinson's, and Alzheimer's. Therefore, detoxifying the liver and gut is essential if you want to keep inflammatory agents out of the rest of your body.

ELIMINATION: CONSTIPATION AND HEALTH

The importance of elimination to overall health is grossly neglected by most doctors. Many people tell me that their doctors have said that daily bowel movements aren't necessary. This is false. Daily elimination is essential, and two to three movements a day is best. The optimal transit time for food to go from your mouth out through your rectum is twenty-four hours. Yet, in my seventeen years of practice, I have found that the majority of people have transit times that range between forty-eight and seventy-four hours. Looking at this on a larger scale, we see a nation that is suffering from an epidemic of constipation, irritable bowel syndrome, and colitis.

The main cause of all these conditions is inadequate water and fiber intake from fresh fruits, vegetables, and whole grains. When grains are refined, both minerals and fiber are stripped away, robbing the body of nourishment and the assistance the fiber provides in cleaning the colon walls.

If your bowels are backed up, your GI tract must focus more on getting rid of waste than on absorbing nutrients, which sets the stage for malnutrition and dysbiosis. Elimination problems also cause autotoxicity. Toxins that are not released from your body fast enough are reabsorbed into the bloodstream. Constipation can also make the pH level in the large intestine more alkaline, creating a breeding environment in which yeast, parasites, bacteria, and viruses thrive.

CANDIDA'S IMPACT ON
THE IMMUNE SYSTEM

The last, but most important, area affected by an imbalance in the digestive system is the immune system, which is simply your body's mechanism for identifying self (what naturally belongs in the body) from non-self (foreign material) and using antigens to destroy or neutralize whatever is foreign.

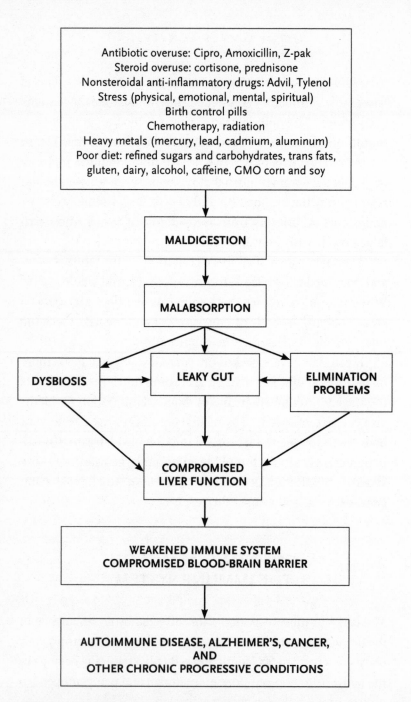

FIGURE 2.2 Digestive Tract and Immunity

The immune system is composed of lymphocytes (B and T cells), the thymus, the spleen, the bone marrow, the lymph nodes, the tonsils, the adenoids, the appendix, the lymphatic vessels, the liver, and Peyer's patches (clumps of lymphoid tissue in the small intestine). This gallant army of organs and cells comes to your rescue whenever foreign invaders attack your body. However, the immune system becomes compromised from chronic maldigestion, malabsorption, leaky gut, intestinal dysbiosis, elimination problems, compromised liver function, heavy metals, medications, stress hormones, and poor diet (see Figure 2.2). This is why a chronically toxic body can give rise to autoimmune diseases in which immune cells, such as the T cells, B cells, and macrophages, mistakenly attack the body's tissues.

ALL BODY SYSTEMS ARE CONNECTED

You can clearly see from what you've just read in this chapter that every organ and system in your body is interlinked. All the systems "talk" to each other. If one organ becomes compromised, another organ will take over and try to compensate. When your gut is leaky, it compromises your bloodstream with toxins. A polluted bloodstream and lymph system compromise your immune system. And an overtaxed immune system allows chronic inflammatory agents to enter your brain, heart, joints, muscles, organs, and so on. The key, then, is to keep toxins moving out faster than they accumulate so that the body stays balanced and healthy over time.

CHAPTER 3

THE CANDIDA
SOLUTION:
A TWO-PRONGED
STRATEGY

Your body has an innate intelligence that allows it to heal itself. You simply need to give it the right environment for a long enough period of time in which to do so. The 90-day protocol I outline in this book provides you with everything you need to create that environment.

The goal of treating candidiasis is to kill fungus and eradicate excess yeast. You never fully rid the body of yeast; you just get the levels back into balance. Achieving this balance requires a two-pronged strategy: first, taking an antifungal supplement to kill the yeast overgrowth, and second, modifying your diet to starve off the excess yeast. The treatment is simple, but it takes diligence, discipline, and consistency on your part to achieve a successful outcome.

WHO NEEDS TO BE TREATED?

The best way to identify whether you have yeast infection is to complete Dr. Crook's questionnaire, work with a practitioner who has experience treating candida, and learn more about the subject. In my office, I examine my clients' responses to Dr. Crook's questionnaire, take an extensive case history, and use a quantum software program to identify imbalances in the body. If a client wishes, a blood test and/or stool test to detect *Candida albicans* overgrowth can also be taken, but I usually discourage doing this.

In my experience, I have found yeast and fungus to be very evasive. They like to hide out in the organs and tissues, and therefore blood and stool tests give inconsistent results. So I suggest you save your money.

There are many unhealthy people whose blood work comes out negative because their conditions are subclinical (undetectable on lab tests), and therefore they end up being misdiagnosed. Their chemistry is often more sensitive than the norm and so even though they are symptomatic, their condition does not show up on a blood test. Also, in general, the blood is often the last system to show signs of imbalance, as the rest of the body will compensate in order to keep the blood levels normal.

For example, when it comes to survival, maintaining the proper blood pH is the body's priority. The body's fluids and tissues have different pH, or acidity level, ranges. Blood needs to be at a pH of 7.35 (alkaline). If the pH varies by even a few tenths of a percent, symptoms will appear, and if it varies by more than one-half of a pH unit, serious illness or death will occur. When the body compensates for a pH imbalance, other tissues and organs in the system may suffer. Your doctor may not even recognize these effects if he's just looking at blood test results.

Be aware that testing the pH of your saliva is different than testing your blood pH, so don't panic if your salivary pH is out of balance.

The money and research that are necessary to develop better functional tests to diagnose candidiasis and other gut imbalances have been lacking because Western medicine has largely failed to recognize the true nature of these problems. Without accurate diagnostic testing, other methods must be used.

In the rare cases in which I do use blood and stool tests, even when the results come back negative, I do not rule out treating the client for candidiasis, as I rely heavily on the other aspects of my evaluation. In fact, in seventeen years of practice and seeing thousands of clients, I have let only a handful of people out of my office without starting them on a candida protocol. That's because using the protocol to first clear infection and inflammation from the client's body allows me to truly discover if there are any other body systems out of balance.

Living as we do in such a toxic world—with stress levels higher than ever—every one of us would benefit from removing infection and inflammation from the body. Even if you have mild symptoms, following the protocol I recommend will help you to experience more energy, greater mental clarity, and an overall sense of lightness within your body.

PREPARING YOUR BODY FOR TREATMENT

You need to be aware that starting a program of food elimination and taking an antifungal can create a Herxheimer reaction (also known as Jarisch-Herxheimer reaction) in which you experience die-off symptoms from killing the yeast. This detoxification process may make you feel worse before you feel better, and you may experience flu-like symptoms, headaches, body aches, abdominal distress, or a worsening of your existing symptoms. To assist with this process, you need to make sure that all your elimination pathways—your kidneys, bowels, lungs, liver, and skin—are functioning optimally. This section will give you a brief overview of what this entails. In Chapter 7, you will find more detail on the nutritional supplements you will be taking to detoxify, support, and strengthen your body as you rid yourself of yeast overgrowth.

Kidneys and Bloodstream

To cleanse your kidneys and blood, as well as your liver and lymph, I recommend drinking red clover tea. This herb helps move the detoxification process along more quickly. Slowly work up to drinking one quart (four eight-ounce cups) of the tea (hot or cold) daily. See Chapter 7 for directions on making the tea. Do not drink this tea, however, if you have grass allergies, ulcers, or acid reflux, or if you are taking blood-thinning medication. Instead, drink one to two cups of dandelion root tea daily.

Red clover tea does not contain caffeine, but it may initially keep some people awake at night because it stimulates the movement of waste out of the body, which can cause insomnia. If you are affected in this way when drinking the tea at night, finish your last cup by no later than 5:00 p.m.

If your die-off symptoms are too intense, you will need to cut down on your dosage of the antifungal remedy and red clover tea. Slowly increase the amounts again as you feel better. Stick with the program and work with your practitioner. Die-off symptoms usually mean that you're on the right track because toxins are coming out into the bloodstream. Reactions might include fatigue, headaches, and possibly a worsening of your existing symptoms, which is why you need to increase your detoxifying supplements slowly. These initial symptoms usually pass within a couple of days to a week.

It's important to realize that there's a difference between an allergic reaction and a die-off reaction. With an allergic reaction, you will experience hives, swelling of the throat, or intense itching of the body. If you experience any of these symptoms, discontinue the antifungal, all supplements, and the tea. Wait three days to allow your body to calm down and then reintroduce the antifungal, each supplement, and the tea, one at a time. Observe your body for two days before adding in another supplement or the tea. If you react severely again, discontinue that supplement or tea altogether.

To keep balanced, it is important to drink enough fluids in the form of water and herbal tea. Drink one-half your body weight in ounces of water and tea, which should include the four cups of red clover tea for cleansing purposes. For example, a 150-pound person needs to drink 75 ounces of water and tea a day.

Bowels and Elimination: Keeping Things Moving

A daily bowel movement is essential; two to three times a day is ideal. Even if you are consuming adequate amounts of fiber in fruits and vegetables and are eliminating daily, I recommend taking added fiber in the form of organic ground flaxseed. It not only assists you to eliminate each day but also removes the toxins, such as mucous, yeast, and other debris, that have built up on your colon walls. Take one tablespoon daily, either in water or sprinkled on salads or vegetables. Fiber in the form of flaxseed meal can be used indefinitely. Avoid products that contain psyllium (unless you have diarrhea) because it can create more gas and bloating.

If you are still constipated after using flaxseed, you can add an herbal stimulant. See Chapter 7 for other supplements that can help with this problem.

Lungs and Breathing

Seventy-five percent of the toxins you eliminate will leave your body through your respiration. To assist with the release of toxins, take at least ten deep breaths each waking hour.

Lymph and Skin

Sweating and stimulating the lymph system are essential for moving waste out of the body. Dry, steam, and infrared saunas are a great way to help the skin and lymph system release toxins.

Dry skin brushing is a simple yet effective way to stimulate the lymph system. Purchase a natural fiber, long-handled brush from your local health food store. Before getting into the shower, brush your skin, starting with the soles of your feet and brushing with short gentle strokes upward toward your heart. There is no need to brush your skin hard. Lymph fluid sits right under the surface of the skin, and therefore it is more effective to brush gently. Brush up your legs, up your back, and then over your shoulders down to the heart (center of your chest). Brush up your arms to the heart. Do not brush your face, as the bristles can scratch facial skin. You may be able to handle soft strokes from the neck down toward your heart. Brush for a total of three to five minutes.

Another excellent way to cleanse the body is with an ionic foot spa, a cylinder-shaped unit that you put into a footbath filled with water (see Resources at the back of the book). The ionic spa produces positively and negatively charged particles, or ions (through the electrolysis of water), that are absorbed through the skin. This can improve cellular functioning and boost energy throughout the body, making it easier for cells to purge toxins. I suggest using this unit once every ten days.

The most important thing you can do to detoxify your lymph and skin is exercise. Exercise stimulates the lymphatic system and skin to move toxins out of the body more effectively. Brisk walking, swimming, isometric exercises, qigong, yoga, and even marching in place while you watch your favorite television show are all good forms of exercise.

Gallbladder and Liver

Lastly, your liver and gallbladder must effectively excrete chemicals and toxins from the body. When you do a candida cleanse, years of toxins will be stimulated to release from your body.

The bile—the emulsifying fluid stored in the gallbladder that helps break down fats, carry toxins from the liver, and stimulate peristaltic action of the bowel—can become thick and muddy after years of indulging in cheese, trans fats, and sugar. Therefore, for the first month of your candida protocol, I recommend a gallbladder decongestant. Gallbladder abX by Quintessential Healing, or Lipogen by Metagenics are products I suggest. Start with one capsule daily with food, slowly increasing the dosage every two to three days until you get to one capsule three times a day.

For the second and third months, you want to go deeper by

supporting the liver. Look for products that will help the liver to conjugate chemicals and make them water soluble so they are excreted from your body rather than recirculated. I suggest Liver abX by Quintessential Healing, or Daily Liver Support by ReNew Life. Slowly work Liver abX up to one capsule three times a day with food, just as you did with the Gallbladder abX.

TAKING AN ANTIFUNGAL

The antifungal supplement you take is crucial. It can be either herbal or pharmaceutical. Herbal antifungals are safer, while many of the pharmaceuticals are harsh on the liver. Be aware that getting your doctor to prescribe a pharmaceutical antifungal can be challenging. If you are turned down, don't waste time trying to get a prescription—herbal antifungals are just as effective and safer for the body, and it's easy for you to get started with them on your own.

Herbal Antifungals

Herbal antifungals are readily available. You can find many of them at your local health food store, on Internet warehouse sites such as www.vitacost.com, or at a health practitioner's office. In my practice, I have found the following to be the most effective for my clients:

- Candida abX (Quintessential Healing, Inc.)
- Candida Cleanse (Rainbow Light)
- Pau d'arco (lapacho): liquid tincture, pills, or tea

These remedies have antifungal properties that target yeast overgrowth and also contain substances that are antiparasitic, antibacterial, and antiviral.

If you cannot find any of these products (see Resources), look for yeast-eliminating products at your health food store that contain one or a combination of some of the following ingredients:

- Pau d'arco (lapacho)
- Citrus seed extract
- Oregon grape root
- Oregano oil
- Black walnut
- Garlic
- Ginger
- Berberine sulfate
- Gentian root
- Undecylinic acid
- Marshmallow
- Caprylic acid
- Fennel

Pharmaceutical Antifungals

The pharmaceutical antifungals include Nystatin, Diflucan (fluconazole), Nizoral (ketoconazole), Sporonex (Itraconazole), and Lamisil (terbinafine). These are a good choice if you have an autoimmune disease, mental illness, or cancer. While herbal antifungals are effective, they are not as concentrated as pharmaceuticals, and so with severe health conditions a pharmaceutical can create faster changes. If you decide to go the pharmaceutical route, you need to find a physician to prescribe them and educate you on the effects of these drugs. My recommendation would be to use Nystatin and/or Diflucan, as I have seen this help many of my clients.

Nystatin: Nystatin is a concentrated extract of a soil-based organism that works by directly killing the yeast. It comes in pill or liquid form. Do not take Nystatin liquid; it contains sugar, which will only feed yeast.

As the authors of *The Yeast Syndrome* state: "Nystatin is virtually nontoxic and nonsensitizing. All age groups, including debilitated infants, accept the drug without demonstrating major side effects, even on prolonged administration."[1]

Nystatin is not initially well absorbed into the bloodstream, but with prolonged use it does get into the blood and thus helps those with autoimmune diseases and cancer. The problem is that most doctors prescribe Nystatin for less than six weeks. Results are better if usage continues for three months or longer. When I was treating myself for MS, I took Nystatin for three years.

Diflucan (fluconazole): Diflucan is a synthetic antifungal drug that is effective against systemic candida overgrowth. It is ten times stronger than Nystatin but also more toxic to the liver. If you use Diflucan or any other systemic antifungal (Nizoral, Sporonex, or Lamisil) for more than a week, make sure to have your doctor test and monitor your liver enzymes.

If you have symptoms of severe depression and/or anxiety, a mental illness, autoimmune disease, or cancer, you can use Diflucan to jump-start the eradication of the fungus. I suggest taking Diflucan (150 mg) for a limited time only, three pills total, one pill every three days, and then switching to an herbal antifungal such as Candida abX or to Nystatin because they are safer. Also, Diflucan primarily targets the candida in the blood, whereas Nystatin permeates the areas of the GI tract, where yeast overgrowth usually originates. To cure candidiasis, it is essential to tackle both the blood and the gut.

Warning:
If you are wheelchair bound or bedridden, Nystatin and Diflucan may be too strong for your body to handle. Because your circulation is compromised, toxins will not move out of your body efficiently, so a probiotic, such as Flora 20-14 by Innate Response, is a safer choice. Before taking any antifungal remedy, make sure that your bowels are moving daily, and work the remedy up very slowly.

CHANGING YOUR DIET

Eating the right foods is your second line of attack against yeast and fungal overgrowth. You will need to eliminate all sugars, dairy products, refined carbohydrates, gluten, corn, and alcohol while you are taking an antifungal. In addition, for the first one to three months you will need to eliminate all yeast and fermented products. Although these foods don't directly feed the yeast, they often create an allergic or sensitivity response, so it is beneficial to eliminate them in the beginning of your treatment program.

If you have a mild case of *Candida albicans* overgrowth, you can expect to feel better in thirty days and fantastic in ninety. People with autoimmune conditions may require from six months to two years of taking an antifungal and following the diet to get the full benefits of the program.

Remember, starving off yeast and fungus requires both taking an antifungal and following the candida-cure diet for a long enough period of time. Trying to do one without the other will not produce positive results. In Chapter 7, I put the components of the diet and the supplement program together so that you have a step-by-step guide to following the 90-day program.

In order to appreciate the benefits of the foods I am suggesting on the candida-cure diet, in the next chapter I will discuss some nutrition basics and how they relate to maintaining balance in your body so that you can successfully eradicate candida.

CHAPTER 4

POOR DIET:
TRASH IN=TRASH OUT

We must eat not only to survive but also to sustain vitality and optimize the functioning of the more than 300 trillion cells that make up our bodies. The digestion of food—as it breaks down into vitamins, minerals, fatty acids, and glycerol—is a complex chemistry, and what we eat can alter that chemistry either positively or negatively. Sadly, the average American diet consists of large amounts of trans fats, refined sugar, refined carbohydrates, corn, gluten, soy, caffeine, alcohol, and processed foods that are filled with chemicals and preservatives. How can your cells thrive on artificial, depleted food? They can't.

It's a mistake to think that junk food will not negatively affect every cell in your body. The equation is very simple: trash in equals trash out. A good diet is one of the most important components of preventive health and healing a diseased body. What you eat can either rebuild or weaken your immune system as well as determine the quality of your aging process. The increasing numbers of people with allergies, diabetes, heart disease, mental illness, autoimmune diseases, and cancers can be attributed in part to eating an unhealthy diet.

Again, a poor diet causes candida overgrowth, and yeast overgrowth creates the most common symptoms people experience today: fatigue, brain fog, anxiety, depression, insomnia, and weight gain. The great news is that you have control over the food choices you make. Once you educate yourself about the problems you're experiencing, you can start to make the necessary modifications—and quickly notice improvements.

THE IMPACT OF A POOR DIET

Let's examine in detail how unhealthy foods and other substances can upset the balance of your body.

Refined Sugar

Refined sugar in any of its forms is one of the most harmful substances you can consume. Sugar depletes the vital vitamins and minerals that you need to sustain yourself and has absolutely no nutritional value. It drains the body and wreaks havoc on the pancreas, which controls blood sugar levels, weakening the immune system. Well-known nutritionist Ann Louise Gittleman states, "There are over sixty ailments that have been associated with sugar consumption in medical literature."[1] Cancer, *Candida albicans*, and human immunodeficiency virus (HIV) all thrive on sugar (see Table 4.1).

When you begin to read labels, you will see that almost every food on the market—from canned goods to breads to salt—contains sugar in some form. Refined sugar is disguised as sucrose, fructose, dextrose, brown sugar, glucose, evaporated cane juice, high-fructose corn syrup, lactose, and maltose.

TABLE 4.1. Fifty-nine Reasons Why Sugar Ruins Your Health

1. Sugar can suppress the immune system.
2. Sugar upsets the minerals in the body.
3. Sugar may cause hyperacidity, anxiety, difficulty concentrating, and crankiness in children.
4. Sugar produces a significant rise in triglycerides.
5. Sugar contributes to the reduction of the body's defense against bacterial infection.
6. Sugar can cause kidney damage.
7. Sugar reduces high-density lipoproteins (HDL).
8. Sugar leads to chromium deficiency.
9. Sugar can lead to cancer of the breast, ovaries, intestines, prostate, or rectum.
10. Sugar increases fasting levels of glucose and insulin.
11. Sugar causes copper deficiency.
12. Sugar interferes with absorption of calcium and magnesium.
13. Sugar can weaken eyesight.
14. Sugar raises the level of neurotransmitters called *serotonin*.
15. Sugar can cause hypoglycemia.
16. Sugar can produce an acidic stomach.
17. Sugar can raise adrenaline levels in children.
18. Sugar malabsorption is frequent in patients with functional bowel disease.
19. Sugar can cause signs of premature aging.
20. Sugar can lead to alcoholism.
21. Sugar leads to tooth decay.
22. Sugar contributes to obesity.
23. High intake of sugar increases the risk of Crohn's Disease and ulcerative colitis.
24. Sugar can cause symptoms often found in people with gastric and duodenal ulcers.
25. Sugar can lead to arthritis.
26. Sugar can contribute to asthma.
27. Sugar can cause *Candida albicans* (yeast infection).
28. Sugar can contribute to gallstones.
29. Sugar can lead to heart disease.
30. Sugar can cause appendicitis.
31. Sugar can lead to multiple sclerosis.
32. Sugar can cause hemorrhoids.
33. Sugar can contribute to varicose veins.

Continued overleaf

TABLE 4.1. (*continued*)

34. Sugar can elevate glucose and insulin responses in oral contraceptive users.
35. Sugar can lead to periodontal disease.
36. Sugar can contribute to osteoporosis.
37. Sugar contributes to salivary acidity.
38. Sugar can cause a decrease in insulin sensitivity.
39. Sugar leads to decreased glucose tolerance.
40. Sugar can decrease growth hormones.
41. Sugar can increase cholesterol.
42. Sugar can increase the systolic blood pressure.
43. Sugar can cause drowsiness and decreased activity in children.
44. Sugar can cause migraine headaches.
45. Sugar can interfere with absorption of protein.
46. Sugar can cause food allergies.
47. Sugar can contribute to diabetes.
48. Sugar can cause toxemia during pregnancy.
49. Sugar can contribute to eczema in children.
50. Sugar can lead to cardiovascular disease.
51. Sugar can impair the structure of DNA.
52. Sugar can change the structure of proteins.
53. Sugar can contribute to sagging skin by changing the structure of collagen.
54. Sugar can lead to cataracts.
55. Sugar can cause emphysema.
56. Sugar can cause atherosclerosis.
57. Sugar can promote an elevation of low-density proteins (LDL).
58. Sugar can cause free radicals in the bloodstream.
59. Sugar lowers the enzymes' ability to function.

Source: Nancy Appleton, PhD, *Lick the Sugar Habit* (Avery Publishing Group, 1996). Used with permission.

The United States is a nation addicted to sugar. In 1890, the average American ate 10 pounds of sugar a year. Today, that figure is between 170 and 200 pounds. Unfortunately, in our society sugar is not just something that tastes good. It has also become an emotional pacifier. Refined sugar may satisfy your psychological needs for a moment, but ultimately it will destroy your body.

Trans Fats (Bad Fats)

The United States is finally recognizing that trans fats, which have already been banned in Denmark and Canada, are major contributors to heart disease and other serious health conditions. Any food that lists "partially hydrogenated" or "hydrogenated" oil among its ingredients contains trans fats. This means that the oil has been heated to a high temperature for the sole purpose of preserving the food product for a longer shelf life.

Trans fats are found in pastries, breads, crackers, processed foods, microwave popcorn, chips, cookies, and margarines. Research has shown that margarines with trans fats—not butter—are the real cause of blocked arteries. These bad fats are poison because they set off an inflammatory response in the body.

Refined Carbohydrates

I call refined carbohydrates, such as white flour, white rice, and refined grains, "glue and goo." These foods include pastries, cookies, muffins, bagels, breads, donuts, and crackers. Refined carbohydrates coat the lining of your gastrointestinal tract and interfere with the process of absorbing nutrients and of eliminating waste. They are irritants that create leaky gut syndrome and ultimately lead to inflammation, allergies, candida, celiac disease, and malnutrition.

Many breads, whether white or wheat, state that they have been enriched with vitamins and minerals, meaning that vitamins and minerals have been added back into the bread. But the truth is that when the flour is bleached and refined, it loses important micronutrients, fiber in particular, which are still lacking after enrichment. Fiber is essential for proper elimination and for keeping blood cholesterol levels down. Refined carbohydrates contribute to the alarming rates of people with constipation, irritable bowel syndrome, and imbalances in blood sugar levels because they convert rapidly to glucose (sugar). This leads to both hypoglycemia (low blood sugar) and diabetes. Also, the bleaching agent used in refined flour, nitrogen trichloride, is poisonous and has been linked to ulcers, schizophrenia, and MS.

Dairy Products

Bovine dairy products (those from cows) are the leading cause of food allergies. Allergies to these products cause sinus problems and gastrointestinal complaints, such as gas, bloating, cramps, gastritis, and diarrhea. Hyperactivity and irritability are common reactions, especially in children. Asthma, headaches, joint and muscle pain, depression, lack of energy, and skin problems are also attributed to dairy allergies.

Lactaid Milk, in which the lactose, or milk sugar, has been removed, was created for those who are lactose intolerant. However, this doesn't solve the problem for everyone who has trouble with milk. There's a difference between being lactose intolerant and having a milk allergy. Most people actually have both conditions. Lactose intolerance means that you lack the enzyme that breaks down lactose. Having a milk allergy means that the body doesn't recognize the milk protein, sees it as a foreign invader, and defends itself by creating an allergic response.

Many in the medical community and advertising industry tell us that drinking milk is the best way to get calcium. Women are especially targeted because of the rising levels of osteoporosis in our country. Yet the fact is that only 30 percent of the calcium in eight ounces of milk is actually absorbed by the body. Pasteurization destroys the enzyme phosphatase. Without phosphatase our bodies cannot use phosphorous, and without phosphorous we cannot assimilate calcium.

The real cause of calcium deficiencies—and osteoporosis—is excessive consumption of high-acid foods, such as animal meats, caffeine, refined carbohydrates, refined sugars, and pasteurized milk and dairy products. Pasteurization and homogenization of cow's milk alter its mineral composition, making it acidic to the body. Eating these acid-forming foods forces the body to leach calcium and other minerals from the rest of the body to buffer the acidity in the bloodstream and maintain an alkaline condition of pH 7.35. Without this protective mechanism, death would result. To maintain that pH balance, the blood robs minerals, which are alkaline, from the body's biggest storehouse of minerals—the musculoskeletal system. In short, consuming dairy products creates exactly the opposite effect that you may be trying to achieve.

Antibiotics and Hormones in Milk

A major factor to consider when deciding whether to ingest dairy products is the use of antibiotics and hormones in raising cows. According to a *Newsweek* article, "Milk is allowed to contain a certain concentration of eighty different antibiotics—all used in dairy cows to prevent udder infections. With every glassful, people swallow a minute amount of several antibiotics."[2] Bovine growth hormone (RBGH), produced through gene splicing to increase milk production, also ends up in milk. These hormones and antibiotics, which are permitted by the government, are creating imbalances in our children as well as in adults. I'm not talking only about milk but also about products made from milk, such as cheese, ice cream, sour cream, and yogurt. The American Dairy Association is spending big bucks to convince you that "milk does a body good," as the billboard says, but I ask you to think again.

Animal Protein

Animal protein in the form of red meat, pork, chicken, turkey, and fish are questionable food sources as well for a variety of reasons. Pork, beef, chicken, and turkey that are not from organically raised animals also contain antibiotics and hormones. These are passed on to consumers and cause hormonal imbalances and yeast overgrowth. Pork contains higher concentrations of parasites because of what pigs are fed and the fact that pigs do not eliminate toxins efficiently. Red meat is more acidic to your body chemistry than chicken and turkey, especially when cooked beyond medium-rare and when eaten with grains, beans, or starchy vegetables. So organically raised chicken and turkey are better choices.

Unfortunately, fish also contain toxins because our oceans have become polluted with heavy metals and chemicals. Shellfish are particularly high in contaminants, as they are bottom feeders and absorb higher concentrations of chemicals and mercury. Stay away from all tuna, as the mercury levels are very high. Fish such as wild-caught salmon, trout, halibut, sole, sardines, and cod are better choices, but even so, finding clean sources for these fish can be a challenge (see Note page 75).

Caffeine

Caffeine, whether in the form of coffee, soda, tea, or chocolate, is acidic and raises blood sugar levels. It stimulates the adrenal glands to release hormones that put the body into an adrenaline-rush response. This increases the heart rate, which releases stored sugar, causing the pancreas to kick out insulin to bring sugar levels back into balance. Overconsumption of caffeine perpetuates this cycle, exhausting the adrenals and the pancreas, whose health we depend on for optimal energy. The rise in sugar also feeds candida overgrowth in the body.

If you do drink coffee after your 90-day program, make sure that it is organic and buy espresso instead of coffee. Nonorganic coffee is the most chemically treated food product in the world, and both organic and nonorganic coffee are more acidic than espresso. Decaffeinated coffee is even worse because of the chemical processing it undergoes. Drink no more than one cup of organic espresso a day to avoid upsetting your adrenal gland function and blood sugar levels.

Alcohol

All alcohol is a neurotoxin that goes directly into the bloodstream, creates an inflammatory response, and depletes vitamins and minerals in your body. Wine, beer, champagne, and sake do more damage to the body because they are high in sugar, which increases blood sugar levels and feeds candida.

While you're on my 90-day program, if there's a day that you decide to indulge in alcohol, it is better to drink vodka because it is distilled and has no sugar compared to wine, beer, sake, or champagne, all of which greatly increase candida overgrowth.

Food Allergens

Food allergies arise when there are imbalances in your gut, such as maldigestion from eating refined, depleted, and processed food. Large quantities of undigested food particles irritating and passing through the lining of the GI tract will cause an allergic reaction in the bloodstream. The most common food allergies are to milk, corn, soy, citrus fruits, chocolate, eggs, nightshade vegetables (eggplant, peppers, potatoes, tomatoes), and gluten. Allergies to even healthy foods, such as certain fruits and nuts, can also arise when your digestive system is out of balance.

Gluten intolerance and celiac disease are increasing at alarming rates. A study published in the *Lancet* states that *Candida albicans* may act as a trigger in the onset of celiac disease in those who are genetically susceptible. There is a protein in *Candida albicans* known as HWP1, whose structure is similar to that of gluten. When a candida infection is present in the gut it can set off an immune system reaction to HWP1, which in turn causes an allergic reaction to gluten.[3]

Several medical researchers have examined the link between gluten sensitivity and neurodegenerative conditions. In a *Lancet Neurology* article entitled "Gluten Sensitivity: From Gut to Brain," Dr. Marios Hadjivassiliou and his colleagues state: "Gluten sensitivity is a systemic autoimmune disease with diverse manifestations. This disorder is characterised by abnormal immunological responsiveness to ingested gluten in genetically susceptible individuals. Coeliac disease, or gluten-sensitive enteropathy, is only one aspect of a range of possible manifestations of gluten sensitivity. Although neurological manifestations in patients with established coeliac disease have been reported since 1966, it was not until thirty years later that, in some individuals, gluten sensitivity was shown to manifest solely with neurological dysfunction."[4] Part of their study revealed a segment of patients who had white matter lesions on the brain or spinal cord that were similar to those found in patients with multiple sclerosis.

White flour, rye, oats (due to cross-contamination), barley, spelt, kamut, triticale, and wheat contain gluten, a protein that is abrasive to the GI tract and can strip the villi. These hair-like projections attached to the intestinal walls help to absorb nutrients and keep the gut clean of yeast and bacteria. In addition, wheat has been hybridized and is subject to a process known as gluten deamidation, in which it is converted to wheat isolates. These are used as binders and emulsifiers in foods, including meat products, sauces, soups, and some beverages. The isolates are more detrimental than the gluten in native wheat and can cause major disruptions in the body.

If you want to know whether you are gluten intolerant and/or are having autoimmune responses, you can contact Cyrex Laboratories (Cyrexlabs.com). Their Antibody Array 3 tests your transglutaminase reactivity, and their Antibody Array 4 lets you know if you have cross-reactivity to foods other than just gluten. There is a strong relationship between transglutaminases (enzymes) testing positive and autoimmune responses. Those who test positive for transglutaminase and/or celiac disease must avoid gluten permanently.

Soy is another food that has been a topic for debate. In America, the market is flooded with genetically modified soy protein foods, processed tofu, and soy protein powders, which may be harmful to your body, as some research has shown. However, if you examine the diets of Asians, you will find that they use fermented soy products, such as miso and tempeh, and in small amounts. Soy in these forms is more digestible and high in essential amino acids and B vitamins. Unfortunately, fermented soy products are not allowed on a candida-cure diet because they can aggravate candida. The only allowable soy on my program is Bragg Liquid Aminos because the soy is unfermented and non-GMO.

A lot of people are allergic to soy and experience gas and bloating when they eat it. If you have this reaction, I recommend avoiding soy products. There are also studies that say large amounts of soy protein can disrupt thyroid function. Because the jury is still out on whether soy is good or bad for you, I feel it is best to stay away from it.

Artificial Sweeteners and Sugar Alcohols

Artificial sweeteners, such as aspartame, acesulfame-K, saccharin, and sucralose, are promoted as an alternative to sugar for people who want to lose weight or eliminate sugar from their diets. But diet sodas and food products that contain these artificial sweeteners are very damaging to the body. The chemicals used to create these sweeteners, or to change the molecular structure of sugar to create them, are known carcinogens. Aspartame, a known neurotoxin, has been linked to neurological symptoms and conditions such as blurred vision, headaches, dizziness, memory loss, numbness, MS, ALS, and Parkinson's disease.

Sugar alcohols, such as erythritol, maltitol, mannitol, sorbitol, and xylitol, are rising in popularity because they are not as damaging to the body as artificial sweeteners. Sugar alcohols are neither sugars nor alcohols. They are carbohydrates with a chemical structure that partially resembles sugar and partially resembles alcohol, but they don't contain ethanol as do alcoholic beverages. They are incompletely absorbed and metabolized by the body and consequently contribute fewer calories than most sugars; however, because they are not fully absorbed they can ferment in the intestines and cause bloating, gas, and diarrhea.

Of the sugar alcohols listed above, I prefer xylitol in small quantities because it is made by our bodies in the metabolism of carbohydrates, it raises oral pH to be more alkaline when ingested, and it is antimicrobial. Commercial xylitol is obtained from corn or the bark of birch trees. I prefer the latter to avoid products made with genetically modified corn. I suggest taking it only in small amounts (under 1 teaspoon, not daily) for two reasons. Xylitol is a carbohydrate, which means it will feed candida if used in large quantities, and although it is obtained from a natural source, it is chemically processed. Any artificial sweetener or sugar alcohol consumed in moderate to large quantities is toxic to the body.

WHAT IS A HEALTHY DIET?

When I give workshops, people frequently ask, "Since so many foods are linked to cancer, what should I eat and drink?" It's true that your body has to adapt more than ever before because of the pollutant overload in our foods, but you don't need to walk around in fear. The body can handle more than you think. Yet there may come a point when your body starts to shut down if you compound the problem by abusing it with poor dietary choices, putting your energy into negative thoughts and emotions, and continually operating at high stress levels.

So, what is a healthy diet? It's one that consists of 60 percent organic vegetables; 20 percent meat and fish that are antibiotic- and hormone-free (meat from grass-fed animals); 15 percent gluten-free whole grains; and 5 percent organic fruits, nuts, seeds, beans/legumes (once or twice a week), and unrefined oils. By adopting a diet of wholesome, unprocessed food and pure water, you can help the healthy cells and tissues of your organs to replicate.

Fruits, vegetables, and plant foods are abundant in phytochemicals, which help prevent cancer and reverse disease. The most important vegetables to consume daily are dark-green, leafy vegetables—spinach, watercress, collard greens, mustard greens, poke greens, turnip greens, dandelion greens, arugula, baby greens, bok choy, kale, etc.—and sprouts. They are filled with vitamins and minerals, especially B6 and magnesium, which are required for your body's many metabolic processes. Cruciferous vegetables, such as broccoli, brussels sprouts, and cauliflower, contain natural compounds that assist with healthy liver function. Raw nuts and seeds contain essential fatty acids needed for the cellular membrane around each cell.

The more we discover about beneficial compounds in whole foods, the clearer it becomes that eating a healthy diet is essential. By doing so, you stop the progression of disease and reduce the amount of supplementation needed to maintain health.

Organic Food

The synthetic pesticides, fungicides, and herbicides used on conventionally grown food, including genetically modified foods, are carcinogenic. While science hasn't fully disclosed all the negative effects that GMO "designer foods" may have on our bodies, they should be avoided because of the toxic chemicals used to produce them. Eighty percent of U.S. wheat, corn, and soy is genetically modified, and GMO corn is the base that we are feeding all our livestock and fish.

You can avoid chemicals and get the best-quality nutrients by supporting certified organic farmers and eating organic fruits, vegetables, meats, and dairy products. These foods are more expensive, but you and your health are worth the investment. Quality outweighs convenience when it comes to healing your body. Be sure to wash all your fruits and vegetables with a little soap and water or a natural fruit-and-vegetable wash, which you can find in the health food store.

Vegetarian Diet

Vegetarians make a number of valid points about the negative aspects of eating meat. It's true, unfortunately, that animals are treated inhumanely and that the use of hormones and antibiotics to raise them is widespread. Yet I find that eating some animal protein each week is the easiest way to keep your body in balance. See the recommendations below about the best kinds of animal protein to eat.

Vegetarianism is a personal choice that only you can make. If you decide to become a vegetarian, or already are one, educate yourself. Most of my vegetarian clients are unhealthy because they're not compensating for the nutrients they are lacking by avoiding meat—such as certain amino acids and B vitamins. Also, I find that their diets often contain excessive amounts of refined carbohydrates and sugar, which deplete vitamins and minerals and feed candida.

Animal Protein

During the digestive process, animal protein breaks down into amino acids, which your body needs for regenerating and repairing cells, tissues, and organs. Therefore, it is important to eat small amounts of animal protein daily. This also helps to keep blood-sugar levels balanced. Consuming animal protein fewer than three times a week will create deficiencies in your body. If you are a vegetarian, become educated about how to balance proteins and carbohydrates, and about which supplements to take to compensate for the protein deficit.

Eating lean animal protein, such as chicken, turkey, and fish, is best in small amounts (2–4 ounces per serving). Eggs are also a good source of protein and are best prepared poached, soft-boiled, sunny-side up, or hard-boiled. When choosing meat, as much as possible, make sure it is from free-range animals who are not given hormones and who are either grass-fed or whose feed is vegetarian and antibiotic- and GMO-free. Free-range chickens are not confined in small cages and may have a little more room to move around than chickens that are raised on factory farms. However, their conditions are not necessarily humane or sanitary and they are often kept in crowded sheds or lots. Ideally, the best meat to eat is from animals who are pasture raised, where they are truly free to roam outdoors. Finding this type of meat, though, can be a challenge, so you will have to do the best you can given your resources.

Red meat contains high concentrations of saturated fat and can increase inflammation in your body, but some body types do well on small amounts. If you do eat it, choose meat from grass-fed animals, such as bison, and eat it only once a week. Listen to your body to feel if you're craving meat. When preparing red meat, cook it rare to medium-rare, as this leaves some active enzymes to help you digest it, and do not eat it with starchy vegetables, beans, or grains because this will make your body acidic. If you are still not digesting the meat well, use a protein digestive enzyme that contains HCl and pepsin.

Avoid all tuna and limit shellfish because of their high mercury levels. All fish contain some heavy metals, yet I feel that their benefit as a good source of omega-3 fatty acids outweighs the negatives. Fish such as wild-caught salmon, trout, halibut, cod, sole, and most other whitefish are acceptable when eaten in moderate quantities. Swordfish, mackerel, shark, tuna, and tilefish are highly contaminated with mercury and should be avoided.

Whole Grains

Whole grains are complex carbohydrates that have not been bleached or stripped of their fiber. They include amaranth, barley, brown and wild rice, buckwheat, corn, kamut, millet, quinoa, oats (gluten-free), rye, spelt, teff, triticale, and whole wheat. Grains contain important B vitamins, which keep your nervous system in balance. They also have fiber to help you eliminate daily and keep your colon lining healthy. The problem is that we eat too much of this food group and only need 25 to 50 grams of carbohydrates a day. After your 90-day program, I recommend living gluten-free and corn-free since they are great aggravators to the body.

Good Fats

As I discussed earlier, there are major differences between good and bad fats. Your body needs good fats such as the omega-3s, omega-6s, and omega-9s because it uses them to coat every cell membrane, and the integrity of the membranes ensures the proper nutrition of your cells. Your body does not manufacture the omega-3 and omega-6 essential fatty acids (EFAs) on its own and only manufactures a limited amount of omega-9s, so you must include them in your daily diet. Good fats help to regulate hormones, blood pressure, heart rate, and nerve transmission as well as reduce inflammation and pain.

Foods high in omega-3 essential fatty acids include deep-sea fish, dark leafy greens, coconut, flax, fish oil, hempseed oil, krill oil, olive oil, raw nuts and seeds, and avocados. Unsalted organic butter contains small amounts of omega-3s as well as vitamins A and D. Even if you consume these foods, you still need to take an omega-3 supplement because you won't obtain enough through your diet. Omega-6 essential fatty acids are found in eggs, grass-fed meat, raw nuts and seeds, and safflower, sunflower, and hemp oils. The best source of omega-9 fatty acids is olive oil, but they can also be found in almonds, avocados, and sesame oil.

Saturated fats from foods such as eggs, coconut meat and oil, butter, ghee (clarified butter), raw goat cheese, and grass-fed meat are beneficial in small quantities. These foods contain important vitamins and minerals, but you should eat them in moderation because large quantities can make the body acidic. Don't be fooled by the claims made about all the low-fat foods on the market and think they are good for you—they contain high concentrations of chemicals and refined sugars, which are unhealthy for your body.

Beans and Legumes

The wide variety of beans and legumes available include adzuki beans, black beans, fava beans, garbanzo beans, kidney beans, lentils, lima beans, mung beans, navy (white) beans, peas, pinto beans, and soybeans. They are high in protein but also high in starch, which converts to sugar in the body. Therefore it's best to eat only small servings so you don't feed candida and cause inflammation. Legumes are also high in lectins (proteins that bind with carbohydrates), which can damage the gut lining and create leaky gut. Adzuki and mung beans are higher in protein than the others, so it's okay to eat slightly larger portions of these. Because of the starch and lectin content, I recommend eating beans and legumes only once or twice a week or skipping them completely for the first two months of your candida-cure diet.

In the U.S. soy is overprocessed and overconsumed and, in most cases, genetically modified. Since there is still much controversy about whether eating it is good or bad for you, I do not recommend eating it in any form, including whole soybeans, tempeh, tofu, soy milk, and soy protein isolate, which is found in protein powder and protein bars. The only soy that is permissible on the candida-cure diet is Bragg Liquid Aminos, which is an unfermented, non-GMO soy sauce.

To remove phytic acid from beans to help with assimilation and avoid flatulence, soak organic beans overnight, discard the water, and cook the soaked beans in fresh water. Prepare beans with one or more of the following herbs and spices for optimal digestion and taste: cumin, clove, caraway, dill, fennel, sage, thyme, onion, oregano, ginger, garlic, rosemary, tarragon, turmeric.

Vegetables

Organic vegetables are loaded with phytochemicals, which your body needs to help it regenerate. Because vegetables have alkalinizing properties, they help reduce acidity in your body, which reduces inflammation. Ideally 60 percent of your daily diet should be vegetables. Green leafy vegetables are nutrient-dense foods and contribute greatly to staying vibrantly healthy, so you need to eat them daily. Because of the nutrient loss in our soils, it is also advisable to take a supplemental green food source (see Chapter 7).

Culinary herbs, such as oregano, thyme, basil, cilantro, parsley, rosemary, and sage, have great healing properties. Make sure to include them in your meals whenever possible.

Lastly, don't forget to incorporate sea vegetables (such as arame, kelp, dulse, nori, wakame, and sea cabbage), which are rich in minerals, including iodine. Most of us are lacking in iodine, which is essential for optimal thyroid function. Sea vegetables also bind with heavy metals and radioactive toxins and move them out of the body.

Fruits

Organic fruits have many beneficial vitamins and minerals that keep your body balanced. You need to limit your intake, though, because fruits are high in natural sugars, which can feed candida. Berries contain the smallest amounts of sugar, and the skins have beneficial antioxidant properties. Limit yourself to one fruit (or a small handful of berries) per day.

Dairy

I have found that after the 90-day program, small amounts of unsalted organic butter and raw goat and sheep products (milk and cheese) are beneficial for supplying the body with amino acids, vitamins, and minerals. Whereas bovine dairy products (from cows) are congesting to the body, goat and sheep products are easier to assimilate because of their molecular structure, which is similar to human milk. Goatein, a product made by Garden of Life, is a high-potency goat dairy powder that is predigested so that lactose-intolerant individuals can consume it.

Think about it—we are the only species that drinks milk from another species. How do cows get their calcium? Not by drinking milk from another species but by eating grass (if they're being raised humanely).

It's more beneficial to get your calcium from organic plant sources than from dairy products, contrary to what the media and most medical doctor's would have us believe. Plant foods that are high in calcium—higher in some cases than cow's milk—include dark-green leafy vegetables, sesame seeds, almonds, broccoli, and carrots. These also contain trace minerals that assist the calcium to enter your bones.

Sweeteners

Acceptable sweeteners for your 90-day program and lifetime are chicory root, luo han guo fruit extract, stevia, and xylitol. Even though xylitol is a carbohydrate, it is metabolized slowly and therefore does not increase sugar levels rapidly. So consuming it in small quantities is acceptable. Make sure your source comes from birch bark (The Ultimate Sweetener from Ultimate Life) instead of corn.

When your candida levels are back in balance after completing the program for 90 days or longer, you might be tempted to go back to the sweeteners you used to indulge in. Be careful, as sugar can bring candida back with a vengeance. Raw, unfiltered honey and coconut nectar in small quantities (once or twice a month) are better choices than evaporated cane juice, agave, brown sugar, etc. Raw honey has amino acids, enzymes, vitamins, and minerals that are beneficial to your body. Coconut nectar has a low glycemic index.

Fermented Foods

I recommend staying off all fermented foods, such as sauerkraut, kefir, cultured vegetables, kimchi, kombucha, tempeh, yogurt, nutritional or brewer's yeast, etc., during your 90-day program. While these do not directly feed candida, as sugar does, fermented foods can initially aggravate a body filled with candida until the gut ecology is more balanced. When you do introduce fermented foods, start slowly and see if they agree with your body.

Raw versus Cooked Foods

Since cooking destroys important enzymes that your body needs for digesting and assimilating foods, the more raw vegetables and fruits you eat, the more enzymes and nutrients your body will take in. However, if your digestive system is out of balance, you might find that initially, for about one to two months, you will do best eating only steamed or cooked vegetables and then gradually increasing your raw food intake with each meal—taking digestive enzymes along with both.

Food Combining

Proper food combining involves eating either protein with vegetables or grains with vegetables but avoiding mixing protein with grains at the same meal. Doing this is beneficial for some people who have digestive problems. Others find that having a little protein along with grains at each meal, whether from an animal or a plant source, keeps both their blood sugar and energy levels more stable. The answer for you lies in listening to your body. If you're hypoglycemic, meaning you have low blood sugar, you'll do best to start off your morning with protein and work your complex carbohydrates into your lunch or dinner meals.

Most people have blood sugar imbalances and do best eating three meals a day plus a snack mid-morning and in the afternoon, as this keeps their metabolism and energy levels balanced. If you are prone to excessive weight loss, however, eat only the three meals a day and avoid snacking in order to slow down your metabolism.

Curing Food Allergies

The best cure for food allergies and intolerances is abstinence. If you suffer from allergies or food sensitivities, eliminate trigger foods for at least one to three months to get rid of allergic reactions. The most common trigger foods are the foods I mentioned earlier: milk, citrus fruits, chocolate, eggs, sugar, nightshade vegetables (tomatoes, peppers, potatoes, eggplant), soy, gluten (barley, kamut, oats, rye, spelt, wheat), and corn. Intolerance reactions may include itchiness, hives, rapid heartbeat, fatigue, constipation, diarrhea, or canker sores.

After a month, you can slowly begin adding trigger foods back into your diet. Your body will tell you if it likes them or not. If your body reacts, you know to stay away from those foods or to eat them in moderation only. Variety is another way to avoid allergic and intolerance reactions. There are plenty of choices in each food group to ensure you are not eating the same thing day after day. As the saying goes, "Eat a rainbow every day."

Water

Our society is dehydrated and, as the eminent researcher F. Batmanghelidj stated, "dehydration is the number one stressor of the human body—or *any* living matter."[5]

How can you keep your body running smoothly when it's

made up of 80 percent water and you drink fewer than eight cups of water a day? You can't. When you do, your "plumbing" gets backed up—your lymphatic system becomes sluggish, your kidneys become overstressed, your colon becomes constipated, and your liver and gallbladder become congested. Autotoxicity occurs as you reabsorb the toxins your body is unable to eliminate. These conditions set the stage for autoimmune diseases and cancer.

Sodas, coffee, iced tea, and fruit juices are not substitutes for water. These do not hydrate the body and its organs in the same way that water does. Batmanghelidj explains that the brain is 85 percent water and says: "Next to oxygen, water is the most essential material for the efficient working of the brain. Water is a primary nutrient for all brain functions and transmission of information."[6] This means that your body needs more water if you are to think and act rationally.

As I said in Chapter 3, the ideal amount to drink is one half of your body weight in ounces of purified or filtered water and herbal tea each day. So if you weigh 150 pounds, you need to drink 75 ounces (or a little over nine eight-ounce glasses) of water daily. To make this easier to do, drink six ounces—a little less than one cup—every waking hour until you go to sleep. If you notice that your urine is a dark in color, this indicates that you are dehydrated. Don't let yourself get to the point of feeling thirsty. Drinking more water can eliminate a number of symptoms, including headaches and pain in the body.

Distilled water is a good choice of drinking water, but it leaches minerals from the body. So if you drink it, make sure to take your vitamin and mineral supplements daily. Sparkling mineral water in small amounts is acceptable as a soda replacement, but only if it's natural and the carbonation has not been added to it. One of the only true natural sparkling mineral waters is Gerolsteiner from Germany.

The best way to ensure that you're getting purified water is to buy your own filtration system. I don't recommend most bottled waters because their manufacturers are not regulated and you don't really know what you're getting. If you do buy bottled water, look for a brand that states on the bottle how the water has been processed, such as through reverse osmosis. If this information is on the label, you have some assurance of the water's purity.

Herbal teas count as water, but because they are also diuretics, you need to make sure to put minerals back in your body by taking your daily multivitamin-mineral supplement. Among the many therapeutically beneficial teas available are red clover, pau d'arco, rosemary, dandelion root, green tea (caffeinated or decaffeinated), chamomile, hibiscus, and mint. Another great hydrator for the body is fresh coconut water, but it should only be drunk after exercising once you have completed your 90-day program, as the average-sized can has 14 grams of sugar in it. You also obtain additional water from eating fresh organic fruits and vegetables.

Juicing

Juicing is a great way to nourish your body. Fresh vegetable juice that has had the fiber extracted will immediately fill your bloodstream with live enzymes, vitamins, and minerals. Juicing is also alkalinizing to your body because it leaches out acidic waste products.

Juicing correctly is important when you are using it as a health treatment. First, don't make more than eight ounces of fresh juice at one time. Drinking large quantities, such as sixteen to thirty-two ounces of carrot juice at one time, can do more harm than good because this is too much sugar for your system.

Second, drink juice on an empty stomach, either an hour before a meal or two to three hours after a meal. Since the juice acts as a treatment for your bloodstream, do not drink it with a heavy meal. Third, drink your juice as soon as you make it. Many of the vitamins and minerals become oxidized within thirty minutes of being exposed to the air. Fourth, drink your juice slowly. Swish it around in your mouth to mix it with your saliva, and then swallow. There are many books on juicing you can use to find recipes that you like. See Chapter 6 for the juice recipe that I recommend most. I recommend the Breville juicer, which can be bought online at www.amazon.com or in many local department stores.

The Vitamix food processor is a wonderful way to eat whole foods and to make soup, but it is different than juicing. A Vitamix keeps the fiber and your digestive system has to break it down, whereas juicing discards the fiber, allowing it to go directly into the bloodstream.

Nutritional Supplementation

In today's world, a good diet alone cannot keep your body healthy. If you want to experience quality aging, your body also requires supplementation. Because modern agricultural practices have depleted our soil, we must eat five times the amount our grandparents ate to obtain the same nutrient value. Our bodies must also cope with more environmental toxicity from pesticides, herbicides, heavy metals, and synthetic chemicals than ever before. On top of that, increased stress levels have weakened our bodies, making supplementation necessary to offset the imbalance.

PART TWO

CREATING YOUR 90-DAY PROGRAM TO BEAT CANDIDA

CHAPTER 5

THE CANDIDA-CURE DIET

N ow that you can better appreciate the nutritional needs of your body, it should be easier to stick to the candida-cure diet, knowing that it will both nourish you and eliminate candida. In a short amount of time, you will recapture your energy and vitality and be convinced that this is the program for you.

The following lists give you general guidelines about the foods that are beneficial to eat and do not promote the growth of yeast, and the foods that you need to avoid because they *do* promote yeast overgrowth. Be aware, however, that everyone's body chemistry is different. Some people have sensitivities or allergies to certain foods on the "Foods to Eat" list, so observe your body in case it reacts negatively to any of the foods. Symptoms such as fatigue, itching, rapid heart rate, gas, burping, bloating, constipation, diarrhea, and headaches are signs that you need to stay away from those particular foods.

Listen to your body. It will tell you what it wants and does not want. Be aware, though, that when your body is toxic, you are going to crave more of the offending foods. But as you cleanse, your body will start to desire healthier foods and it will be easier to trust the signals that it gives you.

You will experience the quickest results within ninety days by adhering to the lists as closely as possible. For those of you who feel you are not able to jump right into the diet, I have included at the end of this chapter a slow-start plan that will allow you to eliminate offending foods gradually and move into the candida-cure diet with greater ease. Your progress, however, will be a little slower, adding about another five weeks to the program.

I have also included in this chapter two weeks' worth of sample menus so you can see that this diet is entirely doable and even enjoyable. You will discover that there are plenty of delicious meals you can easily create. In Chapter 6, you will find recipes for main dishes, side dishes, sauces, desserts, snacks, and beverages as well as a list of the brands I recommend.

FOODS TO EAT

Animal Protein (antibiotic- and hormone-free as much as possible; eat 2–4 ounces daily or no less than 3 times a week)

Beef, bison, lamb (grass-fed; no more than a 3- to 4-ounce serving once a week; prepare rare to medium-rare and eat with greens and not with starchy vegetables, beans, or grains)
Chicken, duck, and turkey
Eggs (organic or pasture-raised, if possible)
Fish (limit shellfish to once or twice a month)

Note: Due to ongoing ocean pollution from many sources, including nuclear leaks at the Fukushima Daiichi power plant in Japan, stay up to date on which fish become contaminated.

Grains (whole and unrefined only)

Amaranth
Breads (gluten-, yeast-, sugar-, and dairy-free)
Brown rice (short and long grain, brown basmati; limit to 2–3 times a week)
Brown rice cakes and crackers (limit to 2–3 times a week)
Buckwheat
Kañiwa
Millet
Oats (gluten-free,* only after 2 months on program)
Pasta (brown-rice, buckwheat, quinoa pasta only; limit to once a week)
Quinoa
Sorghum (can make like popcorn)
Tapioca
Teff
Wild rice
Yucca

Vegetables

All (except corn, mushrooms, peas, and potatoes)
Sweet potatoes, yams, and winter squash (limit to 2–3 servings a week total)

*Oats do not contain gluten; however, they are sometimes cross-contaminated with other gluten grains. Therefore, when eating oats, purchase a brand that ensures that it is gluten-free, such as Bob's Red Mill.

Note: Limit or avoid nightshade-family vegetables for the first 3 months (eggplant, tomatoes, and peppers) because they can cause inflammation. If you eat them and your symptoms increase, avoid completely for the first 3 months and then reintroduce in small amounts if you wish.

Beans and Legumes

You may eat small quantities once or twice a week only or avoid this group entirely for the first 2 months of the program because of their potential to cause inflammation and their high starch levels, which raise blood sugar. If you avoid them and then reintroduce, eat only small amounts once or twice weekly. In either case, do not eat any soy, fermented soy products, or peas. Bragg Liquid Aminos is the only soy product allowed and may be used from the beginning of your program.

Nuts and Seeds (raw; unroasted if commercial; may dry-roast your own)

Almonds
Brazil nuts
Chestnuts
Chia seeds
Flaxseeds
Hazelnuts
Hempseeds
Macadamia nuts
Nut butters (almond and macadamia only; may be raw or dry-roasted)
Pecans
Pine nuts
Pumpkin seeds and pumpkin-seed butter
Sesame seeds (also raw tahini butter)
Sunflower seeds and sunflower-seed butter
Walnuts

Note: Limit quantities of nuts and seeds to a small handful at a time, and chew thoroughly.

Oils (cold-pressed only)

Almond oil (can be used for cooking)
Avocado oil (can be used for cooking)
Coconut oil (can be used for cooking)
Flaxseed oil (not for cooking)
Grapeseed oil (can be used for cooking)
Hempseed oil (not for cooking)
Olive oil (can be used for cooking, low heat only)
Pistachio oil (not for cooking; after 3 months)
Red palm fruit oil (can be used for cooking, low heat only)
Sesame oil (can be used for cooking)

Safflower oil (can be used for cooking)
Sunflower oil (can be used for cooking)
Walnut oil (not for cooking)

Note: At restaurants, eat what is served; be more stringent when using oils at home.

Dairy (antibiotic- and hormone-free only)

Butter (small amounts, unsalted, preferably organic from grass-fed cows)
Clarified butter (ghee, organic)
Goat cheese (raw;* small amounts after 3 months)
Sheep cheese (raw;* small amounts after 3 months)

Fruits† (organic; no dried fruit or fruit juices)

Apples (only sour green apples for first 3 months)
Avocado‡
Blackberries (discard if you see any visible mold)
Blueberries (discard if you see any visible mold)
Coconut flesh and/or unsweetened milk (no coconut juice or coconut water)
Cranberries (fresh, unsweetened)
Grapefruit
Lemons, limes‡
Olives (without vinegar or preservatives only)
Raspberries (discard if you see any visible mold)
Strawberries (discard if you see any visible mold)

Condiments

Apple cider vinegar (raw, unfiltered only—refrigerate)
Bragg Liquid Aminos (unfermented soy sauce; only acceptable soy product)
Dill relish (made without vinegar only; Bubbies; after 3 months)
Dry mustard (or small amounts of mustard made with apple cider vinegar)
Fresh herbs (basil, parsley, etc.)
Himalayan salt
Kelp flakes (Bragg Organic Sea Kelp Delight Seasoning)
Mayonnaise (see Recipes)

*Pregnant and nursing women should not eat raw dairy products.

†Limit fruit intake to one piece per day, about the size of a medium apple in volume, or a handful of berries.

‡Avocado serving and lemon or lime juice may be in addition to your one fruit per day.

Pepper
Rice vinegar (unseasoned and unsweetened only—refrigerate)
Sea salt
Spices (without sugar, MSG, or additives); favor ginger and turmeric
    (anti-inflammatory)

Beverages

Bragg Apple Cider Vinegar Drinks (Ginger Spice, Limeade, and Sweet
    Stevia only)
Herbal teas (red clover, peppermint, green, etc.)
Suja Lemon Love (lemon juice drink)
Unsweetened almond, coconut, and hemp milk
Unsweetened mineral water (Gerolsteiner)
Water (filtered, purified, or distilled only)

Sweeteners

Chicory root (Just Like Sugar)
Lo han (luo han)
Stevia (Kal liquid)
Xylitol (small amounts; The Ultimate Sweetener, Xyla)

Miscellaneous

Cacao powder (raw, unsweetened; small amounts after 2 months)
Carob (unsweetened; small amounts after 2 months because it is an
    inflammatory legume)
Cocoa powder (unsweetened; small amounts after 2 months)
Coconut butter (organic)
Dill pickles (made without vinegar only; Bubbies; after 3 months)
Gums/mints (sweetened with lo han, stevia, or xylitol)
Salsa (without sugar or vinegar, except apple cider vinegar)
Sauerkraut (made without vinegar only; Bubbies; after 3 months)

Foods to Avoid

Avoid the foods on this list while you are on the candida-cure diet. After three months (unless a different time period is specified), you may include the foods below marked with an asterisk (*). Add one food at a time every third day and see if your body reacts—i.e., rapid heartbeat, itching, bloating and gas, constipation, fatigue, or worsening of your symptoms. If this happens, keep these foods out of your diet for another three months and then try again if you wish.

Animal Protein

Bacon (except turkey bacon without nitrates and hormones; gluten-free)
Hotdogs (except chicken and turkey hotdogs without nitrates and hormones; gluten-free; small amounts because high in sodium)
Pork
Processed and packaged meats
Sausages (except chicken and turkey sausages that are gluten-, hormone-, antibiotic-, and nitrate-free)
Tuna (all: toro, albacore, ahi, etc., including canned)

Grains

Barley
Breads (except gluten-, dairy-, yeast-, and sugar-free, but not containing the grains listed here)
Cereals (except gluten-, dairy-, and sugar-free)
Corn (tortillas, polenta, popcorn, chips, etc.)
Crackers (except gluten-, dairy-, yeast-, and sugar-free; do not eat any with corn, potato, and/or white flour)
Farro
Kamut
Oats* (use gluten-free after 2 months)
Pasta (except those made from brown rice, buckwheat, and quinoa)
Pastries
Rye
Spelt
Triticale
White flours
White rice

Wheat (refined)
Whole wheat

Vegetables

Corn
Mushrooms
Peas*
Potatoes

Beans and Legumes

You may eat small amounts once or twice a week or avoid these entirely for the first 2 months of the program because of their potential to cause inflammation and their high starch levels, which raise blood sugar. If you avoid them and then reintroduce, eat small amounts once or twice a week only, but continue to stay off soy (tofu, soybeans, tamari, and ponzu sauce), fermented soy products (miso, tempeh, etc.), and peas.

Nuts and Seeds

Cashews*
Peanuts, peanut butter
Pistachios*

Oils

Canola oil
Corn oil
Cottonseed oil
Peanut oil
Pistachio oil*
Processed oils and partially hydrogenated or hydrogenated oils
Soy oil

Dairy

Cheeses (all, including cottage and cream cheese)
Buttermilk
Cow's milk
Goat's milk and cheese* (raw okay after 3 months, small amounts)
Ice cream
Margarine
Sheep cheese* (raw okay after 3 months, small amounts)
Sour cream
Yogurt

Note: Pregnant and nursing women should not eat raw dairy products.

Fruits

Apricots*
Bananas*
Cherries*

Cranberries (sweetened)
Dried fruits (all, including apricots, dates, figs, raisins, cranberries, prunes, etc.)
Guavas*
Grapes*
Juices (all, sweetened or unsweetened)
Kiwis*
Mangoes*
Melons*
Nectarines*
Oranges*
Papayas*
Peaches*
Pears*
Pineapples*
Plums*
Persimmons*
Pomegranates*
Tangerines*

Beverages

Alcohol
Caffeinated teas (except green tea)
Coffee (caffeinated and decaffeinated)
Energy drinks (e.g., Red Bull, vitamin waters)
Fruit juices
Kefir
Kombucha
Sodas (diet and regular)
Rice and soy milks

Condiments

Gravy
Jams and jellies
Ketchup
Mayonnaise (see Recipes)
Mustard (unless made with apple cider vinegar; small amounts)
Pickles
Relish
Salad dressing (unless sugar-free and made with apple cider vinegar or unsweetened rice vinegar)
Sauces with vinegars and sugar
Soy sauce, ponzu, and tamari sauce
Spices that contain yeast, sugar, or additives
Vinegars (all, except raw, unfiltered apple cider vinegar and unsweetened rice vinegar—keep refrigerated)
Worcestershire sauce

Sweeteners

Agave nectar (Nectevia)
Artificial sweeteners, such as aspartame (Nutrasweet), acesulfame K, saccharin, and sucralose (Splenda)
Barley malt
Brown rice syrup
Brown sugar
Coconut sugar/nectar
Corn syrup
Dextrose
Erythritol (Nectresse, Swerve, Truvia)
Fructose, products sweetened with fruit juice
Honey (raw or processed; raw honey may be used medicinally)
Maltitol
Mannitol
Maltodextrin
Maple syrup
Molasses
Raw or evaporated cane juice crystals
Sorbitol
White sugar
Yacon syrup

Miscellaneous

Cacao/chocolate* (unless sweetened with stevia or xylitol; small amounts after 2 months)
Candy
Carob* (unsweetened, small amounts after 2 months because it is an inflammatory legume)
Cookies
Donuts
Fast food and fried foods
Fermented foods* (kimchi, kombucha, sauerkraut, tempeh, yogurt, nutritional yeast, cultured vegetables, etc.)
Fruit strips
Gelatin
Gum (unless sweetened with stevia or xylitol)
Jerky (beef, turkey)
Lozenges/mints (unless sweetened with lo han, stevia, or xylitol)
Muffins
Pastries
Pizza
Processed food (TV dinners, etc.)
Smoked, dried, pickled, and cured foods

SAMPLE MENUS

The two weeks' worth of sample menus that follow will give you an idea of the diverse menus you can create while on the candida-cure diet. You will find recipes for the starred (*) dishes in the Recipes section, which also includes recipes not listed here. Be aware that some of these meals contain foods and ingredients that you may only eat after being on the diet for two or three months, so familiarize yourself with the "Foods to Eat" and "Foods to Avoid" lists.

WEEK ONE

Day One

Upon arising	1 cup of red clover tea
Breakfast	Poached egg with side of sautéed vegetables (onions and kale), topped with slices of avocado
Snack	Apple (green) with a small handful of raw almonds
Lunch	Amaranth Tabouli*
Snack	Vegetable Alkalizer Juice* (8 ounces)
Dinner	Salmon with dill-lemon juice
	Baby greens salad with Italian Vinaigrette Dressing*

Day Two

Upon arising	1 cup of red clover tea
Breakfast	Vegetable hash (diced onions, spinach, parsnips, and fresh herbs sautéed in olive oil)
Snack	Blueberries topped with coconut butter
Lunch	Wild rice and vegetable stir-fry (see Chicken Stir-Fry recipe)

Snack	Jicama slices dipped in Zesty Tahini Sauce*
Dinner	Tuscan Roast Chicken*
	Artichoke* with melted butter
	Sautéed squash in olive oil and herbs

Day Three

Upon arising	1 cup of red clover tea
Breakfast	Cold cereal (Qi'a Superfood – Chia, Buckwheat & Hemp, original flavor) with berries, unsweetened almond, coconut, or hemp milk and lo han, stevia, or xylitol to sweeten
Snack	Cut-up raw vegetables (broccoli, carrots, jicama, asparagus) with Ranch Dressing*
Lunch	African-Style Turkey*
	Spinach, red onion, and sprout salad with Italian Vinaigrette Dressing*
Snack	Handful of Spicy Almonds*
	1 cup of red clover tea
Dinner	Kelp noodles or quinoa pasta with garlic, pine nuts, basil, and vegetables

Day Four

Upon arising	1 cup of red clover tea
Breakfast	Cinnamon Buckwheat Hot Cereal
	with 1 tbsp ground flaxseed, raspberries, cinnamon, and a splash of almond milk
Snack	Vegetable Alkalizer Juice* (8 ounces)
Lunch	Chicken fajitas with sautéed vegetables, guacamole, and salsa on a lettuce wrap or brown rice tortilla
Snack	Olive Tapenade* on flax crackers
	1 cup of red clover tea
Dinner	Vegetable soup with quinoa

Day Five

Upon arising	1 cup of red clover tea
Breakfast	Egg sandwich (sunny-side-up egg on lettuce wrap with Healthy Mayonnaise,* sprouts, avocado, and sesame seeds)
Snack	Celery sticks with sunflower-seed butter 1 cup of red clover tea
Lunch	Sweetened Butternut Squash* Arugula, Beet, and Walnut Salad*
Snack	Vegetable Alkalizer Juice* (8 ounces)
Dinner	Cod with Macadamia Cream Sauce* Sautéed brussels sprouts and black kale and/or collard greens

Day Six

Upon arising	2 cups of red clover tea
Breakfast	Blueberry-Strawberry Pancakes*
Snack	Green apple with almond butter
Lunch	Quinoa Medley* Cucumber Salad
Snack	Kale chips 1 cup of red clover tea
Dinner	Ground turkey burger (with mustard, baby greens, avocado, and sautéed onion) wrapped in lettuce leaf Side of sliced raw broccoli and cucumbers with Zesty Tahini Sauce*

Day Seven

Upon arising	2 cups of red clover tea
Breakfast	Vegetable scramble with diced squash, cauliflower, mustard greens, chives, and cooked quinoa

Snack	Guacamole with cut-up vegetables
Lunch	Seared halibut salad with Ginger-Wasabi Dressing*
Snack	Tahini Toast*
Dinner	Cornish Game Hen* stuffed with wild rice Side of steamed spinach
Dessert	Baked Apple* with cinnamon

WEEK TWO

Day One

Upon arising	2 cups of red clover tea
Breakfast	Protein Smoothie*
Snack	Half a grapefruit
Lunch	Trout with Ginger-Wasabi Dressing* Grilled asparagus with toasted sesame seeds Citrus Soda*
Snack	Half an avocado with a sprinkle of sea salt 1 cup of red clover tea
Dinner	Quinoa Burger* Asian Coleslaw*

Day Two

Upon arising	2 cups of red clover tea
Breakfast	Rice Almond Pancakes*
Snack	Vegetable Alkalizer Juice* (8 ounces)
Lunch	Chicken Soup*
Snack	Celery and carrot sticks with Ranch Dressing* 2 cups of red clover tea
Dinner	Fish Curry* over brown basmati rice Marinated Kale Salad*

Day Three

Upon arising	2 cups of red clover tea
Breakfast	Arugula and tomato salad topped with grilled onions, turkey bacon, and poached egg, drizzled with olive oil, sea salt, and pepper
Snack	Cucumber slices and sprouts with raw apple cider vinegar
Lunch	Indian Risotto*
Snack	Pumpkin seeds (small handful) 2 cups of red clover tea
Dinner	Turkey Meatloaf* Mashed Faux-tatoes* Side salad

Day Four

Upon arising	2 cups of red clover tea
Breakfast	Qi'a Superfood cereal with almond, coconut, or hemp milk, topped with berries and sliced almonds, and sweetened with xylitol or stevia
Snack	Flax crackers with pumpkin-seed butter
Lunch	Spaghetti Squash with Parsley Pesto Sauce*
Snack	Green apple with small handful of walnuts 2 cups of red clover tea
Dinner	Roast Duckling* Leeks and Leaves*

Day Five

Upon arising	2 cups of red clover tea
Breakfast	Hard-boiled egg with squirt of Basiltops dairy-free pesto
Snack	Handful of Spicy Almonds*

Lunch	Mixed baby-greens salad topped with baked vegetables (peppers, asparagus, zucchini, and yellow squash tossed in olive oil with fresh thyme, sea salt, and pepper)
Snack	Handful of blackberries 2 cups of red clover tea
Dinner	Halibut with Olive Tapenade* Shredded beet and watercress salad sprinkled with toasted pine nuts and Italian Vinaigrette*

Day Six

Upon arising	2 cups of red clover tea
Breakfast	Amazing Meal Vanilla Chai Infusion mixed with 8 oz. of cold unsweetened almond milk
Snack	Jicama with Ranch Dressing*
Lunch	BLT salad (chopped romaine lettuce, diced avocado, cut-up cooked turkey bacon, diced jicama, and Ranch Dressing*)
Snack	Blueberry Buckle Shake* 2 cups of red clover tea
Dinner	Buckwheat soba noodles with vegetables

Day Seven

Upon arising	2 cups of red clover tea
Breakfast	Ground chicken with vegetables (diced cauliflower, peppers, garlic, kale)
Snack	Vegetable Alkalizer Juice* (8 ounces)
Lunch	Wild rice pilaf with sautéed asparagus, purple cabbage, and onions
Snack	Sweet Potato or Parsnip Fries* 2 cups of red clover tea
Dinner	Watercress, fennel, avocado, and sliced green apple salad with Cumin Vinaigrette*
Dessert	Pumpkin Pie*

MEAL IDEAS

The meal ideas below will show you just some of the possibilities for creating tasty meals while on the candida-cure diet. It's important to have a varied selection of foods so you don't get bored with the diet. Limit animal protein to no more than four ounces daily. You will find recipes for the starred (*) dishes in the Recipes section.

Breakfast Ideas

- Eggs or egg whites prepared in a variety of ways with side of steamed spinach, cauliflower, or kale (soft-boiled, poached, hard-boiled, and sunny-side-up eggs are best; eat scrambled or omelets infrequently because of oxidized cholesterol from the yolks, or use egg whites only)
- Soft-boiled eggs with half a grapefruit
- Omelet with vegetables (avocado, spinach, and onion)
- Poached eggs with arugula or spinach: Layer pan with olive oil and large washed handful of spinach or arugula. Crack eggs on top of greens and poach (steam) until yolks are as desired.
- Hard-boiled egg with squirt of Basiltops dairy-free pesto (see www.basiltops.com)
- Egg scramble: Prepare with 2 egg whites, 2–3 spoonfuls of cooked quinoa or wild rice, a few squirts of Basiltops dairy-free pesto, and a handful of washed kale or spinach (sautéed until tender).
- Brown rice tortillas or Sami's Millet & Flax Bread/Lavash with nut butter, coconut butter, or tahini

- Egg sandwich/burrito: poached or sunny-side-up egg, Healthy Mayonnaise,* sliced red onion, and spinach leaves on a heated brown rice tortilla, Sami's Millet & Flax Bread/ Lavash, or lettuce leaf

- Hot cereal (amaranth, brown rice, buckwheat, or quinoa) with nuts, berries, a splash of almond or hemp milk, and sprinkle of cinnamon, sweetened with stevia, lo han, or xylitol if desired

- Turkey bacon or chicken sausage (antibiotic-, hormone- and gluten-free; if casing is pork, peel off after cooking) with sautéed vegetables

- Protein drink made with egg-white, hemp, or rice protein powder (no sugar). Blend with unsweetened almond, coconut, or hemp milk; one piece of fruit from "Foods to Eat" list; handful of spinach or kale; 1 tsp of raw almond butter or coconut oil (melted) or raw nuts/seeds from "Foods to Eat" list; and a couple drops of Kal Pure Stevia liquid (optional).

- Ground turkey or chicken sautéed with diced sweet potatoes and onions

- Cold cereal: Lydia's Sprouted Cinnamon Cereal, Go Raw Simple Granola, or Qi'a Superfood – Chia, Buckwheat & Hemp Cereal (Nature's Path) with almond milk, pecans, berries, and cinnamon, sweetened with stevia, lo han, or xylitol if desired

- Vegetable Alkalizer Juice,* made with organic veggies

- Gluten-free waffles or pancakes, using Namaste Foods Waffle & Pancake Mix: Prepare with unsweetened almond, coconut, or hemp milk (sweeten with stevia, lo han, or xylitol if desired); top with mashed organic berries (blueberries, strawberries, raspberries, or blackberries); and garnish with sliced almonds and cinnamon.

- Amazing Meal Vanilla Chai Infusion (protein drink), mixed with 8 ounces of cold unsweetened almond milk
- Vegetable scramble (arugula, squash, onions, broccoli, and fresh herbs sautéed in olive oil) served over a bed of cooked millet or quinoa
- Leftover dinner from the night before

Lunch and Dinner Ideas

- Salad (greens: spinach, arugula, baby greens, and/or watercress; red onion; sprouts; sliced or grated carrots, jicama, radishes, and/or green apple; nuts, etc.) with Italian Vinaigrette Dressing*
- Black kale salad massaged with fresh lemon juice: Put in refrigerator for a couple of hours to soften kale and then add pine nuts, sea salt, and pepper.
- BLT salad (chopped romaine lettuce, diced avocado, cut-up cooked turkey bacon, diced jicama, and Ranch Dressing*)
- Cruciferous salad (cut-up spinach, watercress, parsley, avocado, red cabbage, green onions, cauliflower, and/or cucumber, topped with sesame seeds and Italian Vinaigrette Dressing*)
- Raw vegetable salad (shredded beets, zucchini, jicama, and chopped cucumber, topped with alfalfa sprouts and dressing)
- Chef's salad (baby greens, tomatoes, and cucumber, with diced cooked turkey, cut-up hard-boiled egg, and dressing)
- Greek salad (romaine lettuce, cut-up cooked chicken breast, olives, and lemon-dill dressing)

- Brown rice and steamed or sautéed vegetables, drizzled with olive oil, Real Salt, and other herbs or spices
- Buckwheat soba or kelp noodles in a stir-fry or with sautéed vegetables or chicken (use cold-pressed sesame oil and Bragg Liquid Aminos)
- Turkey burger with baked Sweet Potato Fries*
- Steamed vegetables topped with Macadamia Cream Sauce*
- Broiled, poached, or sautéed fish (salmon, cod, halibut, sole, trout, etc.) with side of sautéed greens
- Chicken salad on half an avocado
- Stews prepared in a Crock-Pot
- Baked vegetable medley: purple cabbage, kale, onion, red peppers, and brussels sprouts (toss vegetables in olive oil and herbs before baking), served over cooked millet
- Soups, non-dairy and sugar-free (vegetable, chicken vegetable, turkey, leek-broccoli puree, cauliflower-celery, carrot-celery-ginger, parsnip-butternut squash, etc.)
- Brown rice or quinoa pasta with fresh tomatoes, pine nuts, olive oil, garlic, and other vegetables if desired
- BLT wrap (cut-up cooked turkey bacon, lettuce, tomato, and avocado, with small amount of Healthy Mayonnaise*) in brown rice tortilla or lettuce leaf
- Turkey chili with side of mixed green salad (small amounts because of the beans)
- Stuffed zucchini or peppers (ground chicken or turkey, chopped onion, and seasonings) topped with marinara sauce
- Quinoa with vegetables and Basiltops dairy-free pesto

- Chicken or turkey tacos in brown rice tortillas or lettuce leaf, with guacamole, salsa, and shredded lettuce
- Chicken (broiled, roasted, baked, poached) with sautéed kale, cauliflower, and brussels sprouts
- Lamb or beef steak with sautéed onions, with side of sautéed asparagus
- Chicken or turkey sausage cut up and dipped in mustard, with side salad
- Vegetable stir-fry with or without chicken or fish (use cold-pressed sesame oil and Bragg Liquid Aminos)
- Roast chicken prepared with fresh herbs (thyme, rosemary), with side of roasted vegetables (purple cabbage, carrots, peppers, onions, kale—toss veggies in olive oil and seasoning before roasting)
- Turkey dogs (no nitrates, sugar, or dairy) with oven-baked turnip or parsnip fries (toss in grapeseed oil before baking)
- Turkey or chicken sandwich on gluten-, yeast-, dairy-, and sugar-free bread or lettuce wrap, with avocado, spinach, and mustard
- Egg salad sandwich on gluten-, yeast-, dairy-, and sugar-free bread or lettuce wrap (use Healthy Mayonnaise*)
- Lettuce wraps filled with diced chicken salad, wild rice, and slivered almonds
- Cornish Game Hen* stuffed with wild rice, with side cucumber salad (prepared with apple cider vinegar)
- Cabbage rolls stuffed with turkey, pumpkin, and brown rice
- Seaweed wraps filled with wild rice, chopped vegetable medley, and fresh-grated ginger (use organic nori sheets)

Side Dish Ideas

- Shredded slaw salad (raw purple and green cabbage and carrots with rice vinegar and seasonings)
- Collard greens or black kale sautéed in olive oil, with a splash of raw apple cider vinegar
- Sliced cucumbers with apple cider or rice vinegar and sea salt
- Wild rice pilaf made with organic chicken broth (no sugar)
- Mashed sweet potatoes or cauliflower made with almond milk and olive oil
- Artichokes with Dipping Sauce* (melted butter or Healthy Mayonnaise)
- Swiss chard, chopped and sautéed in olive oil, with pine nuts, fresh herbs, and sea salt
- Sautéed onions, peppers, and squashes
- Cold brown-rice salad with raw apple cider vinegar, vegetables, and seasonings
- Parsnips with butter (puree in blender)
- Asparagus sautéed in toasted sesame oil and sprinkled with sesame seeds
- Baked butternut squash with small amount of butter and stevia
- Quinoa with seasonings and spices or Basiltops dairy-free pesto
- Baked brussels sprouts and cauliflower with garlic, sea salt, and olive oil
- Millet with herbs and olive oil or tomato sauce
- Steamed broccoli and cauliflower with melted ghee or butter

- Amaranth with butter and seasonings
- Onions sautéed in olive oil
- Oven-baked turnip fries (toss in grapeseed oil before baking)
- Brown basmati rice sautéed in olive oil with cumin, topped with pine nuts or sliced almonds
- Fresh sprouts (broccoli, alfalfa, radish, sunflower) with fresh lemon juice or raw apple cider vinegar
- Radish and fennel salad with fresh dill and rice vinegar
- Oven-roasted vegetables (squash, onions, carrots, red cabbage) seasoned with thyme and rosemary (toss in olive oil before roasting)

Snacks and Desserts

- Sami's Millet & Flax bread with almond or coconut butter or sesame seed tahini, a drop of stevia, and sprinkle of cinnamon
- Hard-boiled egg with mustard
- Kale Chips*
- Brown-rice cakes or flax crackers with nut/seed butter (almond, macadamia nut, sunflower seed, or pumpkin seed) or coconut butter
- Steve's Original Paleo Stix (grass-fed beef sticks; Steve's PaleoGoods)
- Cut-up vegetables (carrot sticks, broccoli, jicama, celery) dipped in Tahini Sauce,* Ranch Dressing,* or Guacamole*
- Garlic spread (Majestic Garlic) on Jilz Gluten Free Crackerz or on crusts (Mauk Family Farms' Raw Wheat Free or Raw Mineral Rich Crusts)

- Celery with almond butter, macadamia nut butter, sunflower-seed butter, or pumpkin-seed butter
- Fruit from the "Foods to Eat" list, one piece (or a handful of berries)
- Pumpkin or acorn squash slices (baked with olive oil, cinnamon, and sea salt)
- Baked apple with cinnamon and nuts
- Carob or raw cacao muffins (Namaste sugar-free Muffin Mix: add eggs, nuts, berries, unsweetened raw cacao or carob powder, stevia or xylitol (carob and cacao okay only after 2 months)
- Cookies and treats made without gluten, dairy, or sugar (such as Nutty Nibbles by Nut Just a Cookie, sugar-free variety). Or make your own using gluten-free flours; coconut flour; almond meal; butter, ghee, or coconut oil; nut butters; and sweeteners such as stevia, lo han, chicory root, or xylitol.
- Smoothie made with egg-white protein powder, almond milk, blueberries, and nut butter (or melted coconut oil or coconut butter); see Blueberry Buckle shake in Recipes section
- Cacao bars (Rox Chox, made with xylitol; after 2 months)
- DNA Life Bars (after 2 months; made with sweet potato, pumpkin, oats, and xylitol)
- Alchemy Foods Candidly Cookies or Granola

Sauces and Seasonings

- Salsa* (no sugar or vinegar, except raw apple cider vinegar)
- Guacamole* (avocados, tomatoes, onion, and spices)

- Sesame-ginger-garlic sauce, made with cold-pressed sesame oil, ginger, and garlic
- Lemon-garlic sauce, made with olive oil, garlic, and lemon juice (use over gluten-free pasta)
- Fresh-squeezed lemon or lime juice
- Bragg Liquid Aminos (unfermented soy sauce; salty flavor is good for stir-fries)
- Italian Vinaigrette Dressing*
- Unsweetened orange or pineapple juice as a marinade for fish or chicken (these fruits are acceptable only for marinade)
- Healthy Mayonnaise*
- Bragg Organic Sea Kelp Delight Seasoning
- Seaweed flakes
- Curry (coconut milk, turmeric, cumin, ginger, and garlic paste)
- Raw Coconut Aminos (use like soy sauce; www.coconutsecret .com)
- Macadamia Cream Sauce*
- Spices—cayenne, turmeric, ginger, cumin, epazote, coriander, curry, cinnamon, bay leaves, basil, etc.

SOCIAL EVENTS AND
EATING AT RESTAURANTS

You might look at this program and think there's no way you can eat out or go to social gatherings. Sure you can. The key is not to be fanatical. If you are at a restaurant or party and there is barbecued chicken, just scrape off the sauce and eat the chicken, and avoid dipping every bite into the barbecue sauce. If you're at a party and all they're serving is pizza and salad with balsamic vinegar, choose the lesser of two evils—the salad with the balsamic vinegar. If only sandwiches are served, throw away both slices of the bread or eat only one slice.

What will set you back the most—in order of the worst first—are alcoholic beverages, particularly wine, beer, and champagne, because not only are they liquid sugar but they are also fermented, or yeasty. If you indulge in alcohol, drink vodka since it is distilled and has no sugar. Second to set you back is refined sugar—that is, brownies, cookies, pastries, ice cream, etc. Third is dairy, and fourth, white flour products like crackers, pasta, breads, and pizza. With this in mind, it's better to blow it on a piece of cheese than to drink a glass of wine, or to eat pasta instead of a brownie.

Alcohol and sugar do the most damage in setting you back on my program. One trick to help clear your bloodstream when you've eaten something that's not good for you is to drink four cups of red clover tea after indulging. But don't abuse this technique, as you will slow down your progress and not achieve the results you want.

DON'T GIVE UP

Beating candida requires both patience and discipline. If you stick to the diet and supplement program between 80 to 100 percent of the time, you will assure your success. Slipping below 80 percent doesn't mean you won't feel better, but it does mean your progress will be slower.

If you find yourself feeling depressed in grocery stores and restaurants, with their lack of choices of foods you can eat, shop at health food stores and online sites such as amazon.com, vitacost.com, iherb.com, and websites for the product names listed in my book. Not only will you find many wonderful choices but you will also be eating more health-giving, nutritious foods. Wherever you shop, be sure to carefully read labels, as even "health foods" sometimes contain sugar and ingredients you need to avoid while on the candida-cure diet.

It's best to approach getting rid of candida overgrowth as a lifestyle change rather than as a temporary fix. Once you feel better, you'll find that you are more sensitive to how food affects your body and mind, and you won't even want to go back to making poor food choices.

Persevere and the results will come. You'll notice improvements in your health in as little as two to four weeks, and you will experience even greater changes after two to three months. Strict monitoring of your diet is essential. If you continue to eat sugar every day, even in small quantities, you will continue to feed the *Candida albicans* and your progress will be delayed. However, if you've had a "bad day" and eaten something that's not on your diet, don't beat yourself up; just get back on your regimen and keep going.

SLOW-START CANDIDA ELIMINATION FOOD PLAN

Modifying your diet to get healthy can be a challenge. Those who feel they can't immediately jump into the program and adhere to the "Foods to Eat" and "Foods to Avoid" lists can follow a slower candida elimination schedule.

It helps to understand that these dietary changes are not about deprivation—they are about eating foods that will help clear infection and inflammation and restore your health. If you slip up and eat something that's not on the plan, don't let guilt take over. When your emotions get in the way, you're more likely to continue eating foods that are not on the program.

Once you have successfully eliminated all the foods on the following lists, you are ready to begin your first month (Days 1–30) of the 90-day program to eliminate candida and detoxify your body, as outlined in Chapter 7.

Note that some of the foods on these lists may be reintroduced after being on the program for two or three months. Check the "Foods to Avoid" list.

WEEK ONE
Eliminate dairy products
(less dairy = less mucus and inflammation)

Check off items as you eliminate them:

	Check Off
Buttermilk	☐
Cheese (soft and hard)	☐
Cottage cheese	☐
Cow and goat milk (nonfat, low fat, low lactose)	☐
Goat cheese	☐
Ice cream	☐
Margarine	☐
Milk shakes	☐
Protein drinks, powders, or bars that contain dairy ingredients from cows	☐
Sour cream	☐
Yogurt	☐

WEEK TWO
Eliminate refined carbohydrates and gluten
(fewer refined carbohydrates = less inflammation and
greater weight loss)

Check off items as you eliminate them:

	Check Off
Bagels	☐
Barley	☐
Breads with yeast (sourdough, white, buns, rolls, etc.)	☐
Cereals (dry)	☐
Cookies	☐
Corn	☐
Crackers (gluten and white flour)	☐
Donuts	☐
Flour tortillas	☐
Kamut	☐
Oats (gluten-free after 60 days on the program)	☐
Pasta (brown-rice, buckwheat, and quinoa pasta permitted once or twice a week)	☐
Pastries	☐
Pizza	☐
Rye	☐
Spelt	☐
Triticale	☐
Tapioca (except small amounts in brown-rice and teff tortillas)	☐
White flour	☐
White rice	☐
Wheat products	☐

WEEK THREE
Eliminate sugar
(less sugar = less pain and inflammation
and greater weight loss)

Check off items as you eliminate them:

Check Off

Agave nectar (Nectevia) ☐

Artificial sweeteners and sugar alcohols, such as
aspartame (Nutrasweet), erythritol (Nectresse,
Swerve, Truvia), maltitol, mannitol, saccharin,
sorbitol, and sucralose (Splenda) ☐

Barley malt ☐

Brown rice syrup ☐

Brown sugar ☐

Cakes, candy, cereals, chewing gum/lozenges
(except with stevia, lo han, or xylitol), chocolate,
cookies, donuts, ice cream, Jello and gelatins,
pastries, pies, puddings ☐

Coconut nectar/sugar ☐

Corn syrup ☐

Dextrose ☐

Fruit-juice-sweetened products ☐

Fructose ☐

Honey (raw or processed) ☐

Maltodextrin ☐

Maple syrup ☐

Molasses ☐

Soft drinks, soda (including diet soda) ☐

Sucanat, evaporated cane juice crystals,
raw turbinado sugar ☐

Sucralose ☐

White sugar ☐
Yacon syrup ☐

WEEK FOUR
Eliminate miscellaneous foods

Check off items as you eliminate them:

Check Off

Alcohol (even nonalcoholic beers ☐
  because of their yeast content) ☐
Cashews ☐
Coffee (caffeinated and decaffeinated) ☐
Condiments (ketchup, relish, pickles, ☐
  soy sauce, jams, jellies, etc.) ☐
Hydrogenated oils in any food product ☐
  (chips, margarine, breads, etc.) ☐
Kefir ☐
Kombucha ☐
Mushrooms ☐
Peanuts ☐
Peas ☐
Pistachios ☐
Potatoes ☐
All fast foods (hamburgers with buns,
  fried foods, burritos, sandwiches, pizza, etc.) ☐
All fermented foods (miso, tempeh, soy sauce) ☐
All processed foods (TV dinners, bacon, ☐
  beef jerky, bologna, pork sausage, etc.) ☐
All smoked, cured, dried, and pickled ☐
  foods (bacon, bologna, smoked salmon) ☐
Cigarettes and recreational drugs ☐

WEEK FIVE
Eliminate fruits not on "Foods to Eat" list
(less sugar = less inflammation and increased energy)

Check off items as you eliminate them:

	Check Off
All citrus fruits (except lemons, limes, and grapefruit)	☐
All dried fruits (cranberries, dates, figs, raisins, prunes, etc.)	☐ ☐
All fruit juices (sweetened and unsweetened)	☐
All melons	☐
Apricots	☐
Bananas	☐
Cherries	☐
Guava	☐
Grapes	☐
Kiwis	☐
Mangoes	☐
Nectarines	☐
Papayas	☐
Pineapples	☐
Plums	☐
Peaches	☐
Pears	☐
Persimmons	☐
Pomegranates	☐

CHAPTER 6

RECITES

This section will help get you started creating meals that fit within the parameters of your candida-cure diet. You can also experiment with your own ideas, using these recipes as a guideline.

Whenever possible, use free-range, antibiotic-free, and hormone-free beef, chicken, turkey, and eggs. Buy wild-caught fish instead of farmed, and use organic vegetables and fruits whenever possible. Stay away from genetically modified foods. Unless packaged foods specifically state that the product or ingredients are non-GMO or organic, you can assume that they're not. Make sure your mustard is made with apple cider vinegar rather than other types of vinegar, and use purified water for cooking. Whenever a recipe calls for olive oil, use cold-pressed organic extra-virgin olive oil.

Please be aware that some of the recipe ingredients should not be used until you have strictly adhered to the "Foods to Avoid" list for at least two to three months. Xylitol powder (Ultimate Sweetener by Ultimate Life, or Xyla), chicory root (Just Like Sugar), or lo han (Lo Han Sweet by Jarrow) may be substituted for stevia (Kal Pure Stevia liquid) wherever that is called for.

MAIN DISHES

Turkey Quinoa Meatloaf

    1   lb ground organic turkey
    2   eggs
    ¼   cup uncooked quinoa
    1   medium onion, finely chopped
    3   garlic cloves, finely chopped
    2   chilies, finely chopped
    1   tbsp coconut oil or olive oil
    1   tsp thyme
    1   tsp rosemary
    ¼   tsp black pepper
    1   tsp sea salt

Cook quinoa as directed on page 113. Preheat oven to 350°F.
Chop onion, chilies, and garlic cloves finely or in a food processor. Add cooked quinoa and all ingredients to a large bowl and
mix together. Grease a loaf pan with coconut or olive oil, add the
mixture, and bake for 1 hour.

Spaghetti Squash with Parsley Pesto Sauce

    1   medium organic spaghetti squash
    2   cups loosely packed fresh organic Italian parsley, large
        stems removed (don't discard)
    ½   cup roasted macadamia or pine nuts
    2   garlic cloves, minced
    2   tsp lemon juice
    1   tsp lime juice
    ½   cup olive oil
    ½   tsp sea salt
        cilantro, chopped (for garnish)

1. Preheat oven to 375°.
2. Pierce spaghetti squash shell several times with a fork, and place in an oiled baking dish. Bake 25 minutes, turn squash over, and bake until flesh is tender and yields gently to pressure, approximately 20–30 minutes more.
3. While squash is cooking, strip parsley leaves from the stems and set leaves aside. Finely chop the stems and place in a blender or food processor.
4. To make pesto sauce, add the nuts, garlic, lemon and lime juices, oil, and sea salt to blender/food processor and puree. Add the parsley leaves and process until they are coarsely chopped.
5. Once squash is cooked, let cool 10–15 minutes, then cut in half and use a spoon to remove seeds and strings from the center. Gently scrape the tines of a kitchen fork around the edge of the spaghetti squash to shred the pulp into "spaghetti" strands.
6. Put spaghetti into a large bowl, add pesto sauce, and mix well. Sprinkle with chopped cilantro leaves and serve.

Spicy Chicken and Cabbage Soup

   2   tbsp olive oil
   1   large onion, diced
   2   medium carrots, diced
   2   celery stalks, diced
   4   cloves garlic, minced
   8   cups chicken stock (preferably homemade)
   4   chicken breasts, skin removed
  1¾   lbs sauce tomatoes, whole (Roma or dry-farmed Early Girl)
   1   tsp paprika

   1 tsp garlic granules
  ½ tsp dried thyme
  ½ tsp dried oregano
  ½ tsp black pepper
  ½ tsp cayenne pepper
   1 large head green cabbage, cored and coarsely chopped
     Sea salt to taste

Heat the oil in a large stockpot over medium heat. Add onion, carrots, celery, garlic, and a pinch of sea salt. Cook, stirring frequently, until onion is translucent, about 8 minutes. Add chicken stock, chicken breasts, tomatoes, paprika, garlic granules, thyme, oregano, black pepper, and cayenne pepper. Bring to a boil, then reduce heat and simmer, covered, for 20 minutes. Remove the chicken from the pot and strip the meat from the bones. Cut the meat into bite-size pieces. Return the chicken to the pot, add the cabbage, and mix well, breaking up the tomatoes. Add water if the soup is too crowded. Bring to a boil once again. Reduce the heat and simmer, covered, for another 15 minutes. Season with sea salt to taste.

Pico de Gallo Omelet

   4 eggs
     Splash of hemp, almond, or coconut milk
   1 avocado, sliced
   1 cup Pico de Gallo Sauce

Pico De Gallo Sauce

  ¼ cup onion, chopped
   1 large tomato
  ¼ cup cilantro, chopped

Squeeze of fresh lime juice

¼   cup jalapeños, chopped

Beat eggs and milk together. Cook as an omelet. Fill with avocado and Pico de Gallo Sauce.

Cabbage Rolls

1   lb ground white turkey meat

1   tbsp olive oil

¼   cup onion, chopped

¼   cup toasted pine nuts
     Dash of cayenne
     Sea salt and pepper to taste

½   cup fresh tomato, pureed

4–6   green cabbage leaves

8   oz vegetable broth

Rinse and dry cabbage leaves and steam for 3 minutes. While they are cooling, sauté turkey meat, onion, and spices in olive oil until turkey is lightly browned. Add tomato puree and cook over medium heat for about 10 minutes, stirring occasionally. Let cool. Mix in toasted pine nuts. Pour vegetable broth into a baking dish. Fill each leaf with turkey mixture, fold over, and place in the baking dish. Cover with foil and bake at 325° for 30 minutes.

Egg Salad

2   hard-boiled eggs

1   tbsp mayonnaise

¼   cup onion, chopped
     Sea salt and pepper to taste

Mix all ingredients.

Chicken Salad

2   boneless chicken breasts, cubed and baked (without skin)
¼   cup pecans (raw), chopped
½   tsp dill, freshly minced
1½ tbsp mayonnaise
    Sea salt and pepper to taste

Mix all ingredients.

Homemade Chicken Soup

2   large chicken breasts, including bones and skin
1   clove garlic, peeled
1   tbsp olive oil
1   4-oz can of tomato sauce
½   cup carrots, sliced
2   stalks celery, diced (add tops as well for flavor)
1   bunch kale, chopped
1   large yellow onion, chopped
2–3 quarts water
    Sea salt and pepper to taste

Place all ingredients in a 6-quart stock pot. Bring to a boil, and then simmer on low for 3 hours, stirring occasionally.

Fish Curry

1   tsp Thai Kitchen red or green curry paste
1   cup coconut milk, unsweetened
1   tsp fresh lime juice
3   stalks of lemongrass, cut into quarters
1–1½ lbs fresh white fish of your choice, cut into chunks

Combine coconut milk, lime juice, lemongrass, and curry paste in a skillet. Simmer on low for 5 minutes. Add fish. Cook on low for 5–10 minutes. Do not eat pieces of lemongrass, as they are too sharp and chewy.

Chicken Stir-Fry

- 1 tbsp coconut oil
- ½ cup broccoli florets, cut into bite-size pieces
- ½ cup carrots, sliced
- ¼ cup water chestnuts
- 4 oz boneless and skinless chicken tenders, cubed
- ½ cup onion, sliced
- ¾ cup bok choy, chopped
- 1 tbsp Bragg Liquid Aminos
  Toasted sesame seeds

Place wok or skillet over medium heat. Add coconut oil and heat for 3 minutes. Add the rest of the ingredients, except the sesame seeds. Stir-fry on high heat for 5–10 minutes. Cook until vegetables are the desired texture. Top with sesame seeds and serve.

Cornish Game Hens

- 1 cup wild rice, cooked
- 1 tsp olive oil
- ¼ tsp fresh thyme, finely chopped
- ¼ tsp fresh sage, finely chopped
- ¼ tsp fresh rosemary, finely chopped
- ½ cup toasted pine nuts
- 2 Cornish game hens
- 1 onion, peeled and thinly sliced
- 5 garlic cloves, peeled and halved
  Sea salt and pepper to taste
  Butter (melted) and olive oil for basting

Cook wild rice as directed on package to make 1 cup of cooked rice. Mix in olive oil, herbs, and toasted pine nuts. Stuff game hens with rice mixture and place in a roasting pan. Scatter onions and garlic around the outside of the hens. Brush hens with melted butter and olive oil, and season with salt and pepper. Bake at 375° for 1 hour, basting occasionally.

Brown Rice Penne with Chicken Sausage and Vegetables

- 8 oz brown rice penne
- 2 chicken sausage links (peel off pork casings after cooking)
- ½ red bell pepper, diced
- 3 Roma tomatoes, diced
- 1 cup fresh arugula, washed and finely chopped
- 1 tbsp olive oil

Cook brown rice penne in boiling salted water as directed on package. Broil chicken sausage links until cooked. Peel off pork casings when cooled. Slice links and put aside. In a large saucepan, heat olive oil and add bell peppers and tomatoes. Sauté for 10 minutes. Add arugula and cook until wilted. Remove from heat, mix in sliced sausage and penne, and serve.

Quinoa Burger

- 1 medium onion, chopped
- 3 garlic cloves, minced
- 1 tbsp olive oil
- 1 cup cooked black beans
- 1 carrot, finely grated
- ½ cup baked sweet potato (without skin)
- 1 cup cooked quinoa (see recipe below)

1 tbsp caraway seeds
3 tbsp cilantro, chopped
2 tbsp tomato paste
1 tsp raw apple cider vinegar
   Pinch of cayenne (optional)
   Pinch of sea salt

Sauté onions and garlic in 1 tbsp of olive oil. Add beans and cook for 2 minutes. Turn off heat and mash beans in pan. Put beans into a bowl and mix in remaining ingredients. Form patties and bake until heated through, approximately 5–10 minutes on each side.

QUINOA

Soak ¼ cup of raw quinoa for 15 minutes, if possible, to remove the saponin coating, which can have a bitter taste. Rinse quinoa thoroughly. In a saucepan, bring to a boil ½ cup of water, ¼ cup of quinoa, and a pinch of sea salt. Cover and simmer for about 20 minutes. Remove from heat and allow to sit for 5 minutes.

Indian Risotto

1   tbsp ghee (clarified butter)
1   jalapeño, minced
1   tsp cumin seeds
⅛   tsp asafetida
1   cup split yellow mung beans, uncooked
1   cup brown basmati rice, rinsed well in 3 changes of water
1   small cauliflower, cut into florets
6   cups water
½   tsp ground turmeric
1½ tsp sea salt
    Fresh ground pepper to taste

Heat ½ tbsp of ghee in a saucepan. Add jalapeño and cumin seeds. Cook until seeds begin to darken. Add asafetida and stir for a minute. Then add mung beans, rice, and cauliflower, and cook for 3 minutes while stirring. Add 4½ cups of water, turmeric, and salt, and bring to a boil. Lower heat, cover, and simmer, stirring frequently, until the beans and rice are tender (30–40 minutes). Add more water if necessary. Stir in black pepper and drizzle with remaining melted ghee.

Tuscan Country Roast Chicken

  1 roasting chicken, 3 lbs or more, thawed
      Bay leaves to taste (4 fresh or 2 dry)
  ½ lemon (with peel)
      Several garlic cloves, halved
      Sea salt and fresh ground pepper

Preheat oven to 400°. Rinse chicken and wipe dry. Fill cavity with bay leaves, lemon, salt, pepper, and a couple of garlic cloves. Salt and pepper chicken on all sides. Tuck remaining garlic clove halves into the hollows of the thighs and wings. Place chicken on a rack in a roasting pan with about 1 inch of water in the bottom to keep drippings from burning. Bake at 400° for 90 minutes. Reduce temperature to 350° and bake for 15–30 minutes or until legs move easily and juices run clear.

Optional: Make gravy with pan juices, and pour over a whole grain of your choice.

Roast Duckling

  1 4–5 lb duckling, completely defrosted
      Chef's Salt (see recipe below)

4   tbsp butter
1   parsnip or carrot, chopped
2   stalks celery, chopped
1   onion, chopped
2   garlic cloves, thinly sliced
4   black peppercorns
1   bay leaf
½   tsp marjoram

CHEF'S SALT

½   cup sea salt
½   tbsp paprika
½   tsp black pepper
1   tsp white pepper
1   tsp celery salt
1   tsp garlic salt (not powder)

Mix all ingredients for Chef's Salt. Preheat oven to 300°. Spread butter in the bottom of a roasting pan that has a tight-fitting lid. Remove neck and giblets from duck cavity and discard. Rinse duck in cold water and rub inside and out with Chef's Salt. Place duck, breast-side down, directly on the butter in the roasting pan. Place vegetables and garlic inside and around the duckling. Add about 2 inches of water to the pan. Add the peppercorns and bay leaf, and sprinkle marjoram on the duck and in the water. Cover and cook for 2 hours. Carefully remove duckling to a platter and let it cool (if you don't let it cool, it won't turn out right). Split duckling lengthwise by standing it on the neck end and cutting with a sharp knife from the tip of the tail down the center. Quarter if desired. Save leftovers for soup.

Turkey Soup with Winter Vegetables

1 or 2   large turkey legs
2   bay leaves
1   tsp dried parsley
1   tsp dried thyme
1   daikon radish *or*
2   carrots, chopped
1   large parsnip, chopped
2   turnips, chopped
3   stalks celery, chopped
1   yellow onion, chopped
    Sea salt and pepper to taste

Place turkey legs in a large soup pot. Cover with purified water. Add bay leaves, parsley, and thyme and bring to a boil. Simmer for 4 hours, until meat falls off the bones. Strain soup and remove bones. Dice meat and add back into the broth. Add vegetables and simmer for 1 more hour. Salt and pepper to taste.

African-Style Turkey

2   lbs boneless, skinless turkey breasts, cut into bite-size pieces
½   cup chicken or vegetable broth
1   large onion, chopped
4   garlic cloves, minced
½   tsp crushed red pepper flakes
1   tsp fresh ginger, minced or grated
1   tsp sea salt
¼   tsp black pepper
1   tbsp fresh lemon juice

Place all ingredients in a large, covered pot and cook for 45 minutes to 1 hour on low heat. Serve over a whole grain of your choosing.

Marinated Tri-Tip Roast

 1   1½–2 lb tri-tip roast
 ½   tbsp sea salt
 ½   tbsp cracked black peppercorns
 1   tbsp minced garlic cloves
 1   tbsp fresh ginger root, grated
 1   tbsp Bragg Liquid Aminos
 ½   tbsp white pepper
 5   drops of stevia

Mix all ingredients well and cover the meat with them. Place the meat and any excess marinade in a plastic storage bag and put in the refrigerator for at least an hour or, better, overnight. Place meat in a roasting pan and cover it with remaining marinade from the plastic bag. Roast at 425° for 30–35 minutes. When the meat is cooked to desired doneness, carve across the grain into thin slices.

SIDE DISHES

Mashed Faux-tatoes

 1   large head of cauliflower
 ¾   cup unsalted chicken stock (preferably homemade)
 2   tbsp unsalted butter
     Sea salt to taste

Wash cauliflower and cut into pieces. Combine cauliflower and chicken stock in a 2-quart pan. Bring to a boil and then reduce heat. Simmer, covered, until cauliflower is tender, about 20 minutes. Remove from heat, but do not drain the liquid! Mix the butter in and let it melt. Puree the mixture in the pan using an immersion blender. Add sea salt to taste and mix well again.

Artichokes with Dipping Sauce

1   artichoke per serving
1   bay leaf
    Pinch of sea salt
1   tbsp Healthy Mayonnaise per serving (see page 124)

Wash artichokes. Cut off stems to base and stand upright in a large saucepan. Add 2–3 inches of water to the pan. Add the bay leaf and sprinkle the sea salt into the water. Cover and simmer over medium heat until the base is tender—about 45 minutes. Add more water if needed. Use Healthy Mayonnaise as dipping sauce.

Stir-Fried Asparagus

10–12 spears of asparagus
    4   tbsp olive oil
    3   tbsp sesame oil
    6   garlic cloves, minced
    ½   tsp sea salt
        Crushed red pepper to taste

Heat wok or skillet over medium heat. After 1 minute, add oils and heat for 1 minute. Add asparagus and turn heat to high. Stir-fry for 5 minutes or until asparagus are seared, or lightly browned. Add garlic, salt, and red pepper, and stir-fry for about 2 more minutes. Serve hot.

Broccoli with Sliced Almonds

1 large head broccoli cut into small florets
¼ cup raw sliced almonds
2 tbsp olive oil
Sea salt and pepper to taste

Steam broccoli for 7 minutes. Dry-fry almonds in skillet over low heat for 2–3 minutes; then add olive oil and broccoli. Sauté for 2–3 minutes, adding sea salt and pepper to taste.

Sweetened Butternut Squash

1 butternut squash
1 tbsp butter
⅓ cup chopped pecans or walnuts
Spices to your liking (cinnamon, nutmeg, or pumpkin pie spice)
Pinch of powdered stevia

Cut squash in half. Place cut-side down in a pan with ¼ inch of water. Bake at 375° for 1 hour or until soft. Scoop out desired amount of squash flesh and top with butter, nuts, and spices to taste.

Arugula, Beet, and Walnut Salad

1 large bunch arugula, washed well (discard stems)
¼ cup red onion, chopped
½ cup tomatoes, diced
1 apple, diced
¼ cup beets, cooked and diced
¼ cup walnuts, raw or dry-roasted in 350° oven for 10 minutes
Italian Vinaigrette Dressing (see page 122)

Southern Greens Mix

    2   cups mixed collard greens, chard, and mustard greens
    1   tbsp olive oil
    1   tbsp raw apple cider vinegar
    1   tsp raw, hulled sesame seeds
        Pinch of sea salt

Heat skillet. Add olive oil and heat for one minute. Add kale and sauté over low heat until tender. Add the remaining vegetables and ingredients, and sauté for another 3 minutes.

Marinated Kale Salad

    3–4   cups black kale, shredded
      2   tomatoes, diced
      1   carrot, grated
     ¼   cup red onion, diced
     ½   avocado, diced
         Vinaigrette Dressing

Vinaigrette Dressing

     ¾   cup raw apple cider vinegar
     ¼   cup toasted sesame oil or olive oil
      3   garlic cloves, minced
      1   tsp mustard powder

Toss the kale and vegetables (not the avocado) with the vinaigrette dressing. Marinate for at least 4 hours or overnight in refrigerator so vegetables become tender. Add avocado when ready to eat.

Asian Coleslaw

    2–3   cups cabbage, chopped
     ¼   cup daikon radish, grated

¾ cup green onions, finely chopped
1 green apple, finely chopped
1 cup sliced raw almonds or sunflower seeds
2 tbsp raw, hulled sesame seeds
   Sea salt and pepper to taste
   Coleslaw dressing

COLESLAW DRESSING

¼ cup sesame oil
¼ cup rice vinegar (unseasoned, unsweetened)
2 tbsp fresh lemon juice
1–3 drops of stevia liquid

Put all ingredients in a jar and shake well. Pour over coleslaw mixture. Season with salt and pepper.

Candied Yam

1 small yam
   Butter
1–3 drops of stevia liquid

Bake yam at 350° until tender, about 45 minutes. Slice open and add butter and stevia.

Sweet Potato or Parsnip Fries

2 sweet potatoes or 3 large parsnips, sliced like French fries
2 tbsp grapeseed oil
   Sea salt

Put sliced sweet potatoes (or parsnips) in a bowl. Pour grape-seed oil over them and mix to make sure oil covers all sides. Lay out fries on a baking sheet and sprinkle with sea salt. Bake at

400° for 45 minutes. After 20 minutes, turn fries over to cook on the other side.

Leeks and Leaves

6 leeks
2–3 tbsp butter
½–1 cup vegetable stock (use larger amount if you like a soupier mixture)
1–2 bunches spinach, chard, or kale, or a mixture, chopped
Pinch of nutmeg
Sea salt to taste

Trim the leeks, using only the white and pale green parts. Slice in half lengthwise, wash well, and dry. Slice crosswise into small pieces. Sauté leeks in butter in a large skillet until they soften and begin to fall apart. Add stock and season lightly with sea salt and nutmeg. Stir and simmer for 5 minutes. Add greens and simmer until cooked.

SAUCES, DRESSINGS, AND DIPS

Italian Vinaigrette Dressing

¾ cup olive oil
¼–½ cup raw, unfiltered apple cider vinegar
2 stalks rosemary sprigs
1 cup fresh basil, chopped
3 garlic cloves, peeled and mashed
1 tsp dry mustard (optional)
1–2 drops stevia liquid or ¼ tsp stevia powder (optional)

Put all ingredients in a jar and shake well. Keep refrigerated.

Cumin Vinaigrette

½ cup olive oil
1 tsp Eden Foods Organic Yellow (or Brown) Mustard
½ tsp ground cumin
½ tsp minced garlic
2½ tbsp raw apple cider vinegar

Put all ingredients in a jar and shake well. Keep refrigerated.

Ranch Dressing

1 cup whole, raw macadamia nuts (soak for 1–2 hours; rinse and drain)
½ fresh lemon, squeezed
1 tsp sea salt
1 tbsp fresh chives
1 tsp fresh or dried parsley
1 garlic clove *or* 1 tsp garlic powder
1 tsp fresh dill
¼ tsp black pepper
⅓ cup olive oil
Pinch of cayenne (optional)
Purified water, as needed

Blend all ingredients in blender until smooth. Add enough water to achieve the desired consistency.

Ginger-Wasabi Dressing

1 tbsp ginger, freshly grated
¼ tsp fresh horseradish root, grated
¼ cup rice vinegar, unsweetened
1 tsp sea salt

Healthy Mayonnaise

1   egg
1   tsp Eden Foods Organic Yellow (or Brown) Mustard
1   tbsp raw, unfiltered apple cider vinegar *or* fresh lemon
    juice
¼   tsp sea salt
¾   cup grapeseed oil or sunflower-seed oil

Put the egg, mustard, vinegar or lemon juice, and sea salt in
blender or food processor. Blend until smooth. Slowly add in
oil and pulse until smooth and creamy.

Zesty Tahini Sauce

¼   cup raw tahini
2   drops stevia liquid *or* ¼ tsp stevia powder (optional)
    Purified water and/or fresh lemon juice if needed to
    achieve desired consistency
    Pinch of cayenne

No-Cheese Pesto

3   cups fresh basil
¾   cup olive oil
1   tsp sea salt
4   garlic cloves, peeled
½   cup dry-roasted pine nuts
2   tbsp fresh lemon juice

Blend all ingredients in blender and serve over vegetables or
brown rice pasta.

Olive Tapenade

½   cup black olives, pitted and chopped
3   tbsp fresh lemon juice

1 tbsp olive oil
1 tsp sea salt
¼ cup dry-roasted pine nuts, finely chopped

Hand mix all ingredients.

Guacamole

1 medium-sized ripe avocado, peeled and pitted
4 tsp fresh lemon juice
1 tsp onion, finely chopped
Sea salt to taste
Fresh cilantro, chopped (optional)

Mash avocado and mix in remaining ingredients.

Salsa

2 cups tomatoes, diced
1 tbsp olive oil
1 medium onion, chopped
1 tbsp fresh lemon juice
1 jalapeño, finely chopped
Sea salt and pepper to taste

Hand mix all ingredients.

Macadamia Cream Sauce

15 raw macadamia nuts
½ tsp sea salt
Juice of ½ fresh lemon
¼ cup basil, chopped
1 garlic clove

Blend all ingredients in blender. Add more lemon juice if needed for desired consistency. Use on vegetables and grains.

Tahini Dressing

3   tbsp tahini
1   tbsp raw, unfiltered apple cider vinegar
4   tbsp olive oil or flaxseed oil
3   tbsp fresh lemon juice
2–3 drops stevia
     Seasonings as desired (fresh garlic or garlic powder, sea salt, pepper, pinch of cayenne)

Put all ingredients in a jar and shake well. Keep refrigerated.

GRAINS

Rice-Almond Pancakes

1½ cups brown rice flour
¼   cup almond flour
1   egg
¼   cup almond milk
¼   tsp cinnamon
⅔   cup water
4   drops or ½ tsp stevia
     Dash of vanilla extract (alcohol-free)

Combine all ingredients to desired consistency (more liquid equals thinner pancakes). Butter skillet and cook until golden brown.

Blueberry Muffins

1½ cups Namaste Muffin Mix (sugar-free)
½–1 cup organic blueberries or raspberries
1   tsp baking soda
½   tsp nutmeg

2 tsp cinnamon

1 tsp vanilla extract (alcohol-free)

2 eggs

2 tbsp water

½ cup butter, softened

1½ cup chopped pecans

Heat oven to 350°. Lightly oil muffin tin or insert paper liners. Combine all ingredients in large bowl. Fill tins to top with batter. Bake 14–16 minutes or until toothpick inserted in center comes out clean.

Blueberry-Strawberry Pancakes

2 cups Namaste Foods Waffle & Pancake Mix

2 eggs

2 tablespoons coconut oil, melted

⅛ cup raw sliced almonds

½ cup water or unsweetened almond, coconut, or hemp milk

¼ cup blueberries

Pinch of cinnamon or nutmeg

¼ cup strawberries (wash and cut tops off, mash into a puree with fork, and sweeten with small amount of xylitol or stevia)

Butter or grapeseed oil

Combine eggs, melted coconut oil, nuts, water or milk substitute, blueberries, cinnamon/nutmeg, and Namaste mix, and mix well. Add more liquid if you desire thinner pancakes. Preheat pan with butter or grapeseed oil on low to medium heat. Add batter and cook to desired doneness. Top with pureed strawberries.

Sesame Millet

    1   cup uncooked millet
    3   cups water
    1   tsp sea salt
    2   tbsp olive oil
    ¼   cup raw, hulled sesame seeds

Wash millet and drain. Boil water and add sea salt. Add millet, cover, and simmer on low heat for 25–30 minutes. Let stand for 5–10 minutes to increase fluffiness. While millet is standing, put sesame seeds into a frying pan and toast over low flame for 5 minutes, stirring frequently until golden brown. Once seeds are brown, add olive oil and millet. Stir mixture over medium heat for 5 minutes and serve.

Quinoa Medley

    2   cups uncooked quinoa
    ⅔   cup red bell peppers, finely diced
    5   scallions, finely chopped
    ½   cup dry-roasted pecans, finely chopped
    1   cup (or to taste) Italian Vinaigrette Dressing (see page 122)

Cook quinoa for 10–15 minutes (see cooking instructions, page 113). Drain and let cool. Add peppers, scallions, pecans, and dressing. Stir and serve.

Hot Quinoa Cereal

    1   cup unsweetened almond or coconut milk
    ⅓   cup Quinoa Flakes (Ancient Harvest Quinoa)
        Dash of sea salt
        Frozen organic blueberries, handful
        Liquid stevia

Add quinoa flakes and salt to rapidly boiling milk. Return to boil and cook for 90 seconds, stirring frequently. Remove from heat and allow to cool (cereal will thicken slightly). Add stevia to taste and a handful of frozen blueberries—the heat of the cereal will defrost the blueberries.

Nutty Brown Rice

    1 cup brown basmati rice; rinse well and
       soak for 20 minutes in water
    1 tbsp grapeseed oil
    ½ cup raw pine nuts
    2 tsp ground cumin
    ½ tsp ground cardamom
    2 cups water for cooking
       Sea salt and pepper to taste

Rinse rice thoroughly. In a pan over low heat, combine grapeseed oil, uncooked basmati rice, cumin, and cardamom. Stir frequently for 5 minutes. Add 2 cups of water, sea salt, and pepper. Bring to a boil. Reduce flame, cover, and simmer for 10 minutes. In a separate pan, roast pine nuts over a low flame, stirring frequently until lightly browned. Turn off the flame under the rice and let the rice sit for another 10 minutes over the burner. Mix in pine nuts and serve.

Amaranth Tabouli

    1   cup amaranth, uncooked
   2½ cups water
    1   cup parsley, chopped
    ½   cup scallions, chopped
    2   tbsp fresh mint
    ½   cup lemon juice

¼   cup olive oil

2   garlic cloves, pressed

Rinse amaranth. Put 1 cup amaranth into a pot with 2½ cups of water and bring to a boil. Reduce heat, cover, and simmer for 20 minutes. Let cool. Place rest of ingredients into a mixing bowl, add amaranth, and toss together lightly. Chill for an hour or more to allow flavors to blend.

DESSERTS AND SNACKS

Pumpkin Pie

CRUST:*

½   cup arrowroot powder

¼   cup almond meal flour†

¾   cup amaranth flour

¼   tsp sea salt

½   tsp ground cinnamon

3   tbsp grapeseed oil

3–4   tbsp water

Preheat oven to 400°. Oil a 9-inch pie pan; set aside. Combine dry ingredients and blend well. Combine oil and 3 tablespoons water and blend with fork. Add all at once to flour. Stir only until a ball forms. If ball appears dry and crumbly, add a little more water, one teaspoon at a time, until ball hangs together. (Moisture content of flour varies.) Put the ball in the pie pan and use your palms to flatten it as much as possible. Use your thumbs and the knuckles of your fist to flatten it further and spread the crust as evenly as possibly to fit the pie pan. (The

---

*The pie crust recipe is a slightly modified version of the recipe found on www.bobsredmill.com.

†You can buy this from Bob's Red Mill or make it yourself with a food processor, using blanched almonds.

original recipe reads as follows, but it is nearly impossible to roll this crust: "Pat or roll crust to fit into pie pan. Dough tears easily, but mends easily using extra bits to patch.") Prick with fork. Bake 3 minutes in 400° oven. Remove from oven and set aside. Lower oven temperature to 350°.

PUMPKIN PIE FILLING:

- 2 cups pumpkin pulp*
- 2 eggs
- ¾ cup Just Like Sugar (table-top style)
- ½ tsp sea salt
- 1 tsp ground ginger
- 1 tsp ground cinnamon
- ½ tsp ground cloves
- 1½ cups coconut milk†

Blend all ingredients together in a blender or food processor. Pour into pie crust and bake at 350° for 45–50 minutes or until knife inserted in the middle comes out clean.

Chocolate Ice Cream
(requires ice cream maker)

- ⅔ cup cacao powder
- 1 cup Just Like Sugar (table-top style)
- 2 14-oz cans coconut milk†
- ¼ tsp stevia powder‡
- 1 tsp vanilla extract (alcohol-free)

*Fresh pumpkin (baked or steamed) always tastes better than canned, so use that if you have the time to cook it yourself.

†Use Native Forest brand organic coconut milk because it has a better consistency; it can be purchased from www.vitacost.com.

‡The batter isn't quite sweet enough with only the Just Like Sugar, and using this little bit of stevia will add the extra sweetness without thickening the batter by adding more Just Like Sugar.

Thoroughly mix all ingredients. Cover and refrigerate overnight. Pour the ice cream batter into your ice cream maker and
follow your machine's directions.

Baked Cinnamon Apple

- 1 medium Granny Smith or pippin apple
- 1 tbsp butter, softened
- 1 tbsp cinnamon
    Pinch of nutmeg (optional)

Remove apple core to about ½ inch from the bottom of the
apple. Make the hole about ¾- to 1-inch wide. Blend the cinnamon and butter and spoon it into cavity of apple. Place apple in
a buttered baking pan with about ¼ inch of water and bake at
350° until tender. Sprinkle with nutmeg.

Spicy Almonds, Walnuts, or Pecans

- 1 cup raw almonds, walnuts, or pecans
    Few dashes of cayenne
- 2–4 drops stevia liquid
- ¼ tsp sea salt

Stir all ingredients together. Spread on baking sheet and bake
at 300° for 10 minutes.

Chocolate Nut Cookies

- 1 stick butter, softened
- ¼ tsp stevia powder
- 1 egg
- ½ tsp vanilla extract (alcohol-free)
- ½ cup buckwheat flour
- ½ tsp sea salt
- ½ tsp baking soda

1 cup almond flour
¼ cup raw pecans or walnuts, chopped
½ cup unsweetened cocoa powder

Mix together the first four ingredients in a bowl. Add remaining ingredients in order. Drop tablespoonfuls of batter onto a greased baking sheet and bake 10 minutes at 375°.

Tahini Toast

1 slice bread (Sami's Millet & Flax Bread)
1 tbsp raw tahini
Pinch of cinnamon
Pinch of powdered stevia or drop of liquid

Blend tahini, cinnamon, and stevia, and spread on toasted bread.

Chocolate Pudding

⅓ cup raw organic cacao powder
½ cup Just Like Sugar (table-top version)
1 tsp vanilla extract (alcohol-free)
1 can (14 oz) coconut milk

In a medium mixing bowl, gently stir all ingredients together until the dry ingredients are thoroughly incorporated into the wet ingredients. Whisk with an electric whisk on high speed for 2 minutes. Cover and refrigerate overnight.

Kale Chips

Lacinato kale
Olive oil
Sea salt
Other spices, as desired

Cut or tear small pieces of kale and massage with olive oil, sea salt, and spices. Bake at 250° for 20 minutes. Stir and bake for another 20 minutes.

Sorghum Popcorn

¼ cup Tru-Pop Popping Sorghum
    Drizzle of olive oil
    Himalayan salt

Add a few grains to a tall-sided pot and heat over medium heat. When the first grains pop, add the rest of the sorghum and stir very slowly with a wooden spoon. When popping begins, cover and turn heat down slightly. Continue to move the grains around by gently shaking the pot handle. When popping slows, remove from heat. Drizzle with olive oil and sprinkle with Himalayan salt or other seasonings of your desire. About 60–70% of the grains will pop, but the whole batch is edible.

BEVERAGES

Raspberry Lemonade

¼ cup fresh raspberries
¾ cup freshly squeezed lemon juice
    Lo Han Sweet (Jarrow) to sweeten

Mix in blender, adding water if needed, and serve over ice.

Hot or Cold Cocoa/Cacao Milk

1 cup unsweetened almond milk (plain)
½ tsp vanilla extract (alcohol-free)
1 tsp raw cacao powder or unsweetened cocoa powder
   Stevia or Lo Han Sweet to sweeten

Heat in a pan if you desire it hot.

Hibiscus Mint Cooler (sun tea)

2 quarts water
½ cup hibiscus flowers
½ cup chopped fresh mint leaves

Put hibiscus flowers, mint leaves, and water in glass jar and set outside in direct sunlight to make sun tea. Bring inside after an hour or two. Strain, and chill in refrigerator. Serve over ice.

Chai Latte

Decaffeinated chai tea (hot or cold)
Splash of unsweetened almond milk

Citrus Soda

Sparkling mineral water (Gerolsteiner)
Wedge of fresh lemon or lime
1 drop stevia liquid

Ginger Ale

¾ cup peeled and chopped ginger root
3½ cups water
2 tbsp vanilla extract (alcohol-free)
1 tbsp lemon extract (alcohol-free)
¾ tsp stevia powder
Sparkling mineral water (Gerolsteiner)

Rapidly boil ginger root in water for ten minutes. Strain and place liquid in a jar. Stir in vanilla, lemon, and stevia. Cool and store in the refrigerator. Add sparkling mineral water to desired concentration when serving.

Kale-Ginger Smoothie

5 leaves of Lacinato kale, center stem removed
2 tsp chopped fresh ginger
¼ cup parsley stems and leaves
½ green apple, chopped
   Juice of ½ lemon, freshly squeezed
½ cup water
1 drop stevia liquid (optional)

Blend until smooth.

Vegetable Alkalizer Juice

3 stalks celery
½ small carrot
½ apple, green (no seeds)
½ cucumber
4–5 large handfuls of raw spinach, watercress, chard, dark green lettuces, black kale,* dandelion greens, cilantro *and/or* parsley
1 clove peeled garlic *and/or* 1-inch slice of ginger (optional)

Place ingredients in a vegetable juice extractor. Drink juice immediately on an empty stomach either an hour before a meal or 2–3 hours after a meal. Makes 8 ounces of fresh-squeezed juice.

Lemon-Poppy Seed Shake

2 oz coconut milk (not low-fat), almond milk, or hemp milk (unsweetened)
8 oz purified water

*Limit to 2–3 times a week due to its goitrogenic effect.

¼ tsp natural lemon extract (alcohol-free)
1 tsp poppy seeds
1 tbsp flaxseed oil
2 scoops of egg white protein powder
2 tbsp nut butter (almond or macadamia)

Put all ingredients into a blender and blend.

Blueberry Buckle Shake

6–8 oz coconut milk (not low-fat), almond milk, or hemp milk (unsweetened)
     Handful of fresh or frozen blueberries
1 tsp natural vanilla extract (alcohol-free)
5–10 drops stevia liquid (Kal Pure Stevia liquid)
1 tbsp flaxseed oil
1 scoop protein powder: egg-white, hemp (Living Harvest), or brown rice (Growing Naturals)
   Handful of walnuts *or* 2 tbsp nut butter (almond or macadamia)
1 tsp cinnamon

Put all ingredients into a blender and blend.

Protein Smoothie

6–8 oz almond milk or hemp milk (unsweetened)
1 scoop protein powder: egg-white, hemp (Living Harvest), or brown rice (Growing Naturals)
   Handful of kale or spinach
1 tsp coconut oil *or* 1 tsp almond butter
½ green apple
   Handful of blueberries
   Pinch of cinnamon
   Pinch of xylitol or stevia (optional)

Almond Milk

1   cup blanched almonds
4   cups water (less or more for desired consistency)
⅛   tsp sea salt
1   drop vanilla extract (optional, alcohol-free)
3–4 drops Kal Pure Stevia liquid (optional)

Put all ingredients into a blender and blend. Put in glass jar and refrigerate. Will store for 6 days.

Herbal Teas

There are various herbal teas to choose from, including lavender, mint, rooibos, chamomile, hibiscus, dandelion root, etc. Green, white, and oolong teas are also good choices if your body tolerates caffeine and you drink no more than one or two cups a day. Add stevia, lo han, or xylitol to sweeten if desired.

RECOMMENDED PRODUCT BRANDS

Many of the recipes in this chapter include ingredients that can usually be found in your local health food store. Buying some of these products and keeping them on hand will give you a head start and help make your daily food choices easier. If your store does not carry an item listed below, let them know you are a regular customer and ask them to special order it for you, or go on the Internet and order direct from the company or affiliated sites that sell those products.

PRODUCT	BRAND NAME
Breads (yeast-, gluten-, dairy-, and sugar-free)	
Brown Rice or Black Rice Tortillas	Food for Life
Millet & Flax Bread, Lavash	Sami's Bakery
Broths	
Organic Free Range Chicken Broth and Organic Vegetable Broth	Imagine
Butter	
Organic butter (unsalted)	Horizon
Organic Ghee (clarified butter)	Purity Farms
Goat's milk butter	Liberte
Cereals, Cold	
Candidly Granola	Alchemy Foods
Qi'a Superfood – Chia, Buckwheat & Hemp Cereal (original flavor)	Nature's Path
Simple Granola	Go Raw
Sprouted Cinnamon Cereal	Lydia's Organics

Cereals, Hot

Amaranth, brown rice, oatmeal (gluten-free, after 3 months), teff	Bob's Red Mill
Brown Rice Cream	Erewhon
Cream of Buckwheat	Pocono
Quinoa Flakes	Ancient Harvest

Condiments

Coconut butter	Artisana
Garlic spreads (various flavors)	Majestic Garlic
Guacamole	Trader Joe's, 365 (Whole Foods)
Liquid aminos (unfermented soy sauce and soy-free seasoning)	Bragg, Coconut Secret
Mustard (with apple cider vinegar only)	Trader Joe's, 365 (Whole Foods), Eden Foods Organic Yellow/Brown Mustard
Organic Sea Kelp Delight Seasoning	Bragg
Pestos, dairy-free (spicy and mild)	Basiltops
Sea salt	Celtic Sea Salt, HimalaSalt, The Grain & Salt Society, Real Salt

Oils

Coconut, flaxseed, grapeseed, olive, sesame	Spectrum (or other brands that are cold-pressed or expeller-pressed)

Crackers

Brown Rice Cakes	Lundberg
Brown Rice Crackers	Hol-Grain Crackers

Cracked Pepper and Sea Salt, Mediterranean, and Tuscan Crackerz	Jilz Gluten Free
Flax and herb crackers (read ingredients)	Raw Makery
Flax crackers (raw crisps and crusts)	Mauk Family Farms
Garden Herb, Pesto, Tomato Basil	Two Moms in the Raw
Hot 'n Spicy Jalapeño Crackers, Super Seed Crackers	Mary's Gone Crackers
Pretzels: Chipotle Tomato, Everything	Mary's Gone Crackers
Various crackers (read ingredients)	Awesome Foods
Pizza Flax Snax, Sunflower Flax Snax, Spicy Flax Snax, Simple Flax Snax	Go Raw

Drinks / Water

Apple Cider Vinegar All Natural Drink (Ginger Spice, Limeade, Sweet Stevia)	Bragg
Lemon Love Water	Suja
Mineral water, sparkling	Gerolsteiner
Smart Water	Glaceau

Whole Grains and Flours

Brown rice	Lundberg
Buckwheat, millet, sorghum, & teff flours (organic)	Arrowhead Mills
Gluten-free grains, flours, wild rice	Bob's Red Mill
Pancake and Baking Mix, Almond Meal Flour, Sweet Rice Flour, and Brown Rice Flour	Authentic Foods
Pancake & Baking mix (buckwheat flax; contains small amounts of white rice flour, so use no more than once a week)	The Pure Pantry
Quinoa flour (organic)	Ancient Harvest

Waffle & Pancake Mix, Sugar-Free Muffin Mix, Perfect Flour Blend, Pizza Crust Mix	Namaste Foods

Meats, luncheon (high in sodium; use small amounts)

Organic Roasted Turkey Breast, Herb Turkey Breast	Applegate Farms
Herbed-Roasted Turkey, Peppered Roasted Turkey, Naturally Oven-Roasted Turkey	Diestel Turkey Ranch
Oven-roasted turkey (no salt), uncured turkey salami	Whole Foods Market (in deli case)

Milk Substitutes (almond, hemp, coconut—unsweetened*)

Almond milk, original and vanilla (unsweetened)	Blue Diamond Almond Breeze
Almond milk (organic), original and vanilla (unsweetened)	Pacific Natural Foods
Almond milk, coconut milk	365 (Whole Foods)
Almond & Cashew Cream (unsweetened; after 3 months)	MimicCreme
Coconut Milk (unsweetened)	So Delicious
Organic Coconut Milk Unsweetened	Asian Creations – Thai Kitchen
Organic Coconut Cream, Organic Coconut Milk	Native Forest
Hempmilk, Unsweetened Original	Tempt (Living Harvest)

*Read the labels, as some of these companies make sweetened and unsweet-ened varieties with the same name.

Nuts & Seeds and Nut / Seed Butters

Almond Butter, Sunflower Seed Butter	MaraNatha
Coconut Butter	Artisana
Pumpkin Seed Butter, organic	Jarrow Formulas
Raw nuts, raw or dry-roasted almond butter, macadamia nut butter	Trader Joe's
Raw nuts and nut butters	Whole Foods
Sesame Tahini, organic	Arrowhead Mills
Tahini, organic	Once Again
Sprouted Pumpkin Seeds, Sunflower Seeds, Spicy Seed Mix, Simple Seed Mix	Go Raw

Pasta

Brown rice pasta	Lundberg, Trader Joe's, Tinkyada
Kelp noodles	Sea Tangle Noodle Company
Penne, spaghetti, fettuccine, elbows, etc.	Rizopia Organic Brown Rice Pasta
Quinoa Pasta	Andean Dream

Protein Powders

Amazing Meal Vanilla Chai Infusion	Amazing Meal
Egg-white protein powder	NOW Foods, MRM
Instant Whites Egg White Protein – Plain	Gifted Earth Originals
Hemp Protein Powder, unsweetened	Tempt (Living Harvest)
Protein Energizer Vanilla Shake	Rainbow Light
Rice Protein, plain or vanilla	NutriBiotic
Rice Protein Powder: Vanilla Blast, Original, or Chocolate Power (after 2 months)	Growing Naturals

Salsa

African Hot Sauces — Brother Bru-Bru's

Habanero salsa — Frontera

Mild or hot salsa — Green Mountain Gringo

Mild or hot salsa — 365 (Whole Foods)

Salsa — Tacupeto

Snacks / Treats

Candidly Cookies, Granola — Alchemy Foods

Chocolate Coconut Fudge and Green Apple Cinnamon bars — DNA Life Bars

Kale chips — Brad's Raw Foods, Alive & Radiant Foods

Nutty Nibbles (sugar-free varieties) — Nut Just a Cookie

Rox Chox (cacao with birch xylitol) — Rox Chox

Steve's Original Paleo Stix (grass-fed beef sticks) — Steve's PaleoGoods

Tru-Pop Popping Sorghum — Just Poppin

Sweeteners

Chicory root (Just Like Sugar) — Just Like Sugar Inc.

Lo Han Sweet — Jarrow Formulas

Stevia, liquid and powdered (different flavors) — Sweet Leaf, Kal

SweetFiber (inulin fiber, lo han guo) — Purpose Foods

Xylitol powder (The Ultimate Sweetener, Xyla) — Ultimate Life, Xylitol USA

Vinegar (always keep refrigerated)

Apple cider vinegar (raw and unfiltered) — Bragg, Spectrum

Rice vinegar (unseasoned, no sugar) — Marukan

WHEAT ALTERNATIVES

The following list gives you an idea of the many ways you can enjoy grains and grain substitutes without using wheat, as well as the different forms in which these foods can be found.

ALTERNATIVE	AVAILABLE IN THE FORM OF
Almond	Flour, meal, almond butter
Amaranth	Cereal, flour
Buckwheat	Cereal, flour, noodles, whole groats
Chestnut	Flour
Coconut	Flour
Hazelnut	Flour
Kañiwa	Flour, whole grain
Kelp	Noodles
Legumes*	Flours (black bean, fava bean, garbanzo bean, mung bean, pinto bean, red and green lentil, white bean)
Millet	Flour, whole grain
Oat*	Bran, flour, meal
Quinoa	Cereal, flour, whole grain
Rice (brown)	Bread, crackers, tortillas, rice cakes, whole grain
Sorghum	Flour, whole grain
Teff	Flour, whole grain
White bean*	Flour
Wild rice	Flour, whole grain, rice cakes

*Avoid for first two months.

CHAPTER 7

YOUR 90-DAY
PROGRAM

I t's now time to look at the 90-day protocol in its entirety—
the candida-cure diet plus the supplements you will be
taking. As I have noted throughout these pages, the supplements serve multiple purposes. They replace the missing
vitamins and minerals in foods that have been grown in depleted
soil, they detoxify your body, and they provide you with the
energy and nutrients you need to experience quality aging after
completing the program.

While I have included specific instructions for taking the
supplements, you will need to work in conjunction with your
health-care practitioner to make sure you are meeting your individual needs. You might want to give your practitioner a copy
of my book or photocopies of specific pages so that he or she
can better assist you.

Here are some guidelines to follow as you embark on this
treatment plan:

GENERAL GUIDELINES

- As with any specialized diet or nutrition supplementation program, you should consult your physician or health-care provider prior to starting any of the programs discussed in this book or to taking any new dietary supplements so he/she can identify any potential interactions with other supplements or prescription medications you may be taking and identify any other risks that might be specific to your health or medical conditions.

- Every individual is different, and my protocol is derived from a collective assessment of thousands of clients I have seen over the years. These are suggestions, not a guarantee.

- Women who are pregnant or breastfeeding should only do the candida-cure diet and take a prenatal multivitamin-mineral supplement, vitamin D3, pure-grade fish oil, and probiotics. Check with your health-care practitioner about the amounts to take. When you are finished breastfeeding, you may start implementing the detox and supplement regime.

- Do not start taking an antifungal if you are not moving your bowels at least once a day. This must be corrected before you start the antifungal. See the Supplementation for Additional Needs section, page 166, for supplements you can take for constipation.

- Purchase your supplements from reputable sources, such as a health practitioner, professional supplement companies, health food stores, or online vitamin warehouses such as vitacost.com, iherb.com, or amazon.com. In the Resources section, I have listed sources for purchasing all the supplements outlined in this section. The small amounts of soy in some of the products I recommend are acceptable and usually non-GMO. Supplements sold in drugstores and supermarkets often contain sugar, synthetic dyes, and fillers. Read labels to make sure they say "no added dyes, fillers, sugar, corn, or yeast."

- The abX products are my line of supplements, which I recommend, having used them with good results for many years in clinical practice. They are a possible choice, not mandatory. What matters most is that you address the areas of imbalance that I write about and use quality vitamins/supplements.

- If you live outside the United States, look for comparable products with similar ingredients to the supplements I have suggested by going online and viewing the ingredient labels of these supplements.

- Periodically check my website, www.annboroch.com, for the latest updates on supplement changes that pertain to this section. Some companies change their formulations, or a supplement may no longer be on the market.

- If you experience an upset stomach when taking any of the supplements that are supposed to be taken on an empty stomach, you may take them after meals. If you experience diarrhea from any supplement, stop taking it for three days, and then try taking one pill once a day and see if you tolerate it. If you do, continue to build up slowly. If you do not, discontinue the supplement permanently.

- Remember to drink adequate amounts of water and herbal teas daily—one half of your body weight in ounces.

At first glance, you might feel overwhelmed by making new food choices and taking all of the supplements. To ease into the program, a week before beginning buy groceries and think about your different meal options, including what you can eat in restaurants while you're following the protocol. Order or purchase the recommended supplements for detoxifying and rebuilding your body (see Resources for vendors). By the end of the first week, you will have started to feel better—you will be clearer, have more energy, and find that you are adjusting to the rhythm of your 90-day program.

Note: Those who have chosen to do the slow-start elimination plan will only begin the following 90-day program after eliminating all the foods listed on pages 100–104.

INSTRUCTIONS FOR YOUR 90-DAY PROGRAM

FIRST MONTH: DAYS 1–30

Candida-Cure Diet

- Do not eat sugars, fermented or yeast products, dairy products, refined carbohydrates, corn, gluten, and trans fats, or drink alcohol.
- Follow the "Foods to Eat" (page 75) and "Foods to Avoid" (page 79) lists in Chapter 5.

Antifungal (work up slowly)

Take one of the following antifungals. Choose either an herbal or pharmaceutical antifungal based on your needs (see pages

40–43 for a more in-depth discussion of the pros and cons of the different options):

- Candida abX (Quintessential Healing, Inc.)
- Candida Cleanse (Rainbow Light)
- Pau d'arco (Gaia Herbs–tincture; Pacific Botanicals–tea)
- Nystatin
- Diflucan (to jump-start only; then switch to Nystatin)

As I explained in Chapter 3, pharmaceutical antifungals (Diflucan and Nystatin) are recommended for autoimmune and cancer conditions or if you have severe anxiety and/or depression or mental illness. Diflucan can be taken to give your body a jump-start and kill off systemic fungus at the beginning of your program. After jump-starting with Diflucan, as described below, you can then switch to Nystatin or an herbal antifungal.

How to take herbal antifungal:
If you are taking Candida abX, Candida Cleanse, or pau d'arco in pill form, start with one capsule or tablet per day and slowly increase the dosage by one capsule or tablet every three days until you reach the dose recommended on the chart on page 158. If any of the antifungals bother your stomach when taking them on an empty stomach, switch to taking them after meals.

When taking the pau d'arco as a tincture, start with one dropperful and slowly increase the dosage every three days until you reach the dosage recommended on the chart on page 158. For the tea, start with one cup per day and increase by one cup every three days until you reach three cups.

Note:
- For severe cases of candida overgrowth, I suggest doubling the dose of herbal antifungals to 2 pills 3 times a

day after meals. At this dose you would be getting closer to the potency of Nystatin.

Diflucan and Nystatin are prescription drugs. You would need to find a physician who is willing to prescribe them, and take according to his/her directions. Below is a regimen that I have seen work for other clients, but always follow the advice of your physician.

Suggested way to take pharmaceutical antifungal (Nystatin):
For an adult, dosing of Nystatin is one pill (500,000 units) taken three times a day without food. Take it with food, however, if it upsets your stomach. Work up slowly to the full dose.

Suggested way to jump-start with Diflucan (option for those with cancer, autoimmune disease, or mental illness):
Ask your doctor to prescribe three 150 mg tablets. Take one pill every three days for one week.

After jump-start, switch to Nystatin:
After your jump-start of three Diflucan tablets (one pill every three days), begin taking Nystatin, slowly working your way up to one pill three times a day. Start off with one pill per day, and after three days, increase to one pill twice a day. After another three days, increase Nystatin to one pill three times a day. Continue at this dosage for six to twelve months. For the third month, add probiotics (11-Strain Probiotic Powder, Flora 20-14, Ultimate Flora 15 billion, or Primal Defense Ultra) and take them at a separate time from the Nystatin.

Or

You can switch to an herbal antifungal:
After jump-starting with Diflucan for one week, switch to Candida abX or one of the other herbal antifungals and take as directed for a minimum of twelve months. To get the greatest benefits from the antifungal, switch to another herbal antifungal every two to three months. For the third month, add probiotics (11-Strain Probiotic Powder, Flora 20-14, Ultimate Flora 15 billion, or Primal Defense Ultra) and take them at a separate time from the herbal antifungal.

Notes:
- If you decide to use Diflucan for more than a week, have your doctor monitor your liver enzymes.
- Antifungals can make you feel worse before you feel better. Work your dosage up slowly to allow your system to keep up with the elimination of toxins.
- If you are wheelchair-bound or bedridden, do not take pharmaceutical antifungals. Start by taking probiotics for month one, and then take Candida abX according to the instructions for herbal antifungals above.

Additional Supplements to Take

The following supplements should be taken according to the recommendations that follow.

Intestinal repair formula (1 scoop in 4–6 oz. of water on empty stomach when arising):

These herbal and amino supplement powders contain flavonoids, phytochemicals, and antioxidants to help restore and repair the intestinal lining. It is essential to repair leaky gut, which will reduce inflammation in the body. These formulas may help with acid reflux, heartburn, ulcers, brain fatigue, and reduce sugar and carbohydrate cravings. Take an additional scoop at bedtime if you have heartburn, gastric reflux, numerous allergies, or intense gastrointestinal symptoms.

Brands:
- Repairvite, K-63 (Apex Energetics)
- IntestiNEW (ReNew Life)

Vitamin C (300–700 mg of whole-food source or 3,000 mg daily):

Buy vitamin C that contains a whole-food source or one with mineral ascorbates and/or bioflavonoids. Plain ascorbic acid crystals may irritate your stomach lining and intestines. Spread the dosage throughout the day because your body will absorb only so much at one time. Increase your dose of vitamin C slowly. If you experience diarrhea, cut back your dose. You can take powders with or without food, but it's best to take pills after a meal or snack.

Brands:
- Truly Natural Vitamin C powder (HealthForce Nutritionals)
- QBC Plex (Solaray)
- Super-C Plus, tablets or powder (Dr. Schulze's)

Blood sugar/adrenal formula (1 pill 3 times a day with food):

These herbal-vitamin supplements help balance blood sugar, assist with hypoglycemia (low blood sugar), balance highs and lows of energy throughout the day, and decrease sugar/carb cravings. They can also be used as needed after the 90-day program whenever sugar/carb cravings kick in or hypoglycemic symptoms return. If you are diabetic, during the 90-day program use an insulin-resistance formula instead, such as Glysen or Pancreas Tonic (see below).

Brands:
- Gluco abX (Quintessential Healing, Inc.)
- Bio-Glycozyme Forte (Biotics Research)

Or

Blood sugar formula for prediabetes/diabetes and insulin resistance (1 capsule 3 times a day with food):

These herbal-vitamin supplements assist with high blood sugar (hyperglycemia) and insulin resistance. They can be used long term if needed after the 90-day program.

Brands:
- Glysen (Apex Energetics)
- Pancreas Tonic (Made in U.S.A.)

Gallbladder formula (work up slowly to 1 capsule 3 times a day with food):

These herbal-vitamin supplements stimulate bile secretion, decongest the gallbladder, and help eliminate toxins from the gallbladder and liver. Use for the first month only, and then switch to a liver formula for the second and third months.

Brands:
- Gallbladder abX (Quintessential Healing, Inc.)
- Lipo-Gen (Metagenics)

Notes:
- If your gallbladder has been removed, still use a gallbladder formula to assist with the digestive process.

- If diarrhea or stomach upset occurs, stop taking the gall-bladder formula for three days and then start up again with one pill a day, slowly working back up to three pills a day. If diarrhea occurs again, stop taking altogether and replace with liver formula.

Vitamin E (400 IU daily):

When buying vitamin E, be sure the source is natural. Look for "d-tocopherol" on the label and not "dl-tocopherol," which is synthetic. Also use an E vitamin that has mixed tocopherols and tocotrienols.

Brands:
- E Gems Elite (Carlson)
- familE (Jarrow Formulas)

Notes:
- Do not take vitamin E if you are on blood thinners.
- If you will be having surgery, stop taking vitamin E two weeks before so your blood will clot properly.
- If you begin to bruise easily, reduce your dosage of vitamin E.

Digestive enzymes (1 after each meal, optional):

It's usually a good idea to add digestive enzymes for the first month or two of your program to make sure you're digesting, absorbing, and eliminating properly. If you have trouble digesting animal protein (burping and heartburn), buy an enzyme that contains pepsin and hydrochloric acid (HCl). If you have low blood sugar—your energy is up and down throughout the day, and you feel shaky and crabby if you skip a meal—use a pancreatic enzyme that contains pancreatin, lipase, protease, and amylase. If you're a vegetarian or have mild digestive complaints, use a plant-based digestive enzyme.

Brands:
- Enzy-Gest (a full-bodied digestive/pancreatic enzyme containing HCl, pepsin, pancreatin, lipase, protease, and amylase; Priority One)
- Digest Gold (plant based for vegetarians, Enzymedica)

Ground flaxseed meal:

Put one tablespoon of organic ground flaxseed meal in eight ounces of water or sprinkle on salads or vegetables. Fiber is key to keeping your bowels moving daily, sweeping debris from the colon lining, and lowering cholesterol.

Brand:
- Bob's Red Mill (keep refrigerated after opening)

Red clover tea (work up slowly to four cups daily):

This herb cleanses your bloodstream, liver, and kidneys. One heaping teaspoon of the loose herb makes one cup of tea. To make four cups of the tea, bring one quart of filtered water to a boil, and turn off the heat. Add four teaspoons of the bulk herb to a large French press, add boiling water, let it steep for fifteen minutes, and then slowly push the plunger down. After brewing, you can add ice cubes to make iced tea to drink throughout the day. Make sure to consume whatever amount you make the same day or it will get moldy, even if kept in the refrigerator.

Notes:
- Do not drink red clover tea if you have grass allergies, ulcers, or acid reflux, or if you are taking blood-thinning

FIRST MONTH: DAYS 1–30 SUPPLEMENT SCHEDULE

Supplement	Arising	Breakfast	Lunch	Dinner	Bedtime	After Meal[1]	Empty Stomach
Antifungal (dose depends on which product is used)[2,3]	X		X (1/2 hour before meal)	X (1/2 hour before meal)			X
RepairVite[4]	1 scoop						X
Vitamin C		Dose depends on which product is used				X (pills/powder)	X (powder only)
Gluco abX or Glysen		1	1	1		X	
Gallbladder abX[3]		1	1	1		X	
Vitamin E (400 IU)		1				X	
Digestive enzymes (optional)		1	1	1		X	
Ground flaxseed meal		1 tbsp any time during the day				X	X
Red clover tea[3]		4 cups daily				X	X
Molybdenum (150 mcg, optional)		1				X	

1. After-meal supplements will digest better and make you feel less bloated if you take them right before your first bite of food vs. last bite.

2. Antifungal/antimicrobial: Candida abX, Candida Cleanse, pau d'arco pills, or Nystatin (1 pill 3 times a day), OR pau d'arco tincture or tea (2 dropperfuls twice a day, or 3 cups tea a day). For severe cases of candida, work up to 2 pills 3x/day of Candida abX or Candida Cleanse. Those jump-starting with Diflucan, take one 150 mg tablet every 3 days for 1 week; then switch to an herbal antifungal or Nystatin. Nystatin can be used for up to 2 years for autoimmune diseases. Work up slowly to the full dose of any antifungal. If an antifungal upsets your stomach, take with meal vs. ½ hr. before a meal.

3. Start slowly with this antifungal/supplement/tea: 1 pill or 1 cup for 3 days; then increase to 2 pills or 2 cups for 3 days, and so on. Do not drink red clover tea if you have grass allergies, ulcers, or acid reflux, or if you are taking blood-thinning medication.

4. RepairVite: Mix with 4–6 oz. of water. Take an additional scoop at bedtime if you have heartburn, acid reflux, numerous allergies, or intense gastrointestinal symptoms.

medication. Instead, drink one to two cups of dandelion root tea daily.

- Buy only organic red clover dried herb. Organic bulk suppliers are Mountain Rose Herbs and Pacific Botanicals (see Resources).
- Some people have reported that drinking red clover tea at night keeps them awake. This is due to the cleansing effect on the bloodstream. If you experience this, it is best to finish drinking red clover tea by 5:00 p.m.

Molybdenum—Die-Off Remedy (150 mcg daily, optional):

This is a trace mineral that assists with the breakdown of acetaldehyde—a main by-product of candida. It can help alleviate die-off symptoms such as brain fog, spaciness, headaches, and vertigo. Take as needed until symptoms subside.

Brand:
- Chelated molybdenum (Country Life)

SECOND AND THIRD MONTHS: DAYS 31–90

Candida-Cure Diet

- Do not eat sugars, fermented or yeast products, dairy products, refined carbohydrates, corn, gluten, and trans fats, or drink alcohol.
- Follow the "Foods to Eat" and "Foods to Avoid" lists on pages 75 and 79.

Antifungal

Continue taking your antifungal at the dosage where you left off at the end of the first month. For severe cases of candida, keep dose of Candida abX or Candida Cleanse at 2 pills 3 times a day.

Supplements

Liver formula (work up slowly to 1 capsule 3 times a day with food):

These herbal formulas assist with liver detoxification by converting harmful chemicals into water-soluble substances so they can be easily eliminated in the urine and feces. Use for months two and three of your program. The liver formula replaces the Gallbladder abX or Lipo-Gen you used during the first month.

   Brands:
   - Liver abX (Quintessential Healing, Inc.)
   - Daily Liver Support (ReNew Life)

Omega-3 fish oil gels (1,200–1,500 mg daily with food):

Omega-3 oil is an essential fatty acid that is not manufactured by the body and which helps decrease inflammation, feed brain and nerve cells, and support cardiovascular function. It is important to buy a brand that is free of PCBs (carcinogenic, man-made chemicals used in electrical equipment and industrial processes). The brands that follow are PCB-free.

   Brands:
   - OmegaGenics EPA-DHA 720 (Metagenics)

- Ultimate Omega 3—fish oil gels (Nordic Naturals)
- Elite Omega-3 Gems Fish Oil, Professional Strength (Carlson)

Note:

- Do not take fish oil if you are on blood-thinning medication. If you will be having surgery, stop taking the fish oil two weeks before so your blood will clot properly.

Blood sugar/adrenal formula (1 pill 3 times a day with food):

If you are still experiencing sugar and carbohydrate cravings and/or are hypoglycemic, stay on Gluco abX or Bio-Glycozyme Forte for days 31–90. However, if you feel stabilized, stop taking Gluco abX and switch to Adrenal abX (see page 162) to assist with balancing adrenal function and to give you more energy.

Brands:

- Gluco abX (Quintessential Healing, Inc.)
- Bio-Glycozyme Forte (Biotics Research)

Or

Blood sugar formula for prediabetes/diabetes and insulin resistance (1 capsule 3 times a day with food):

Keep taking Glysen or Pancreas Tonic for days 31–90 if you are diabetic or are still struggling with insulin resistance. These formulas can be used long term if needed after the 90-day program.

Brands:

- Glysen (Apex Energetics)
- Pancreas Tonic (Made In USA)

Adrenal formula (1 tablet 2 times a day with food):

These herbal vitamin supplements balance adrenal function and are useful for relieving fatigue and the effects of high stress. If you are a vegetarian, you can take Adaptocrine or Adrenal Health (see plant-based formulas below).

Brand:
- Adrenal abX (Quintessential Healing, Inc.)

Or

Plant-based adrenal formulas (for vegetarians; 1 pill 2 times a day with food):

These herbal-vitamin supplements are suitable for vegetarians. They assist with relieving fatigue and the effects of high stress and can be used long term if needed after the 90-day program.

Brands:
- Adaptocrine (Apex Energetics)
- Adrenal Health (Gaia Herbs)

Evening primrose oil (1,000 mg daily: 500 mg twice a day—for women only):

This is an omega-6 essential fatty acid that is rich in gamma linoleic acid (GLA), which assists in balancing female hormones and eliminating PMS symptoms.

Brand:
- Evening Primrose Oil (Source Naturals, NOW Foods)

Vitamin C (300–700 mg whole food source or 3,000 mg daily):

Buy a vitamin C that contains a whole-food source or one with mineral ascorbates and/or bioflavonoids. Plain ascorbic acid crystals will irritate the lining of your stomach and intestines. Spread out the dosage through the day because your body will absorb only so much at one time. Increase your dose of vitamin C slowly. If you experience diarrhea, cut back your dose. You can take powders with or without food, but it's best to take pills after a meal or snack.

Brands:
- Truly Natural Vitamin C powder (HealthForce Nutritionals)
- QBC Plex (Solaray)
- Super-C Plus, tablets or powder (Dr. Schulze's)

Vitamin E (400 IU daily):

When buying vitamin E, be sure the source is natural. Look for "d-tocopherol" on the label and not "dl-tocopherol," which is synthetic. Also use an E vitamin that has mixed tocopherols and tocotrienols.

Brands:
- E Gems Elite (Carlson)
- familE (Jarrow Formulas)

Notes:
- Do not take vitamin E if you are on blood thinners.
- If you will be having surgery, stop taking vitamin E two weeks before so your blood will clot properly.
- If you begin to bruise easily, reduce your dosage of vitamin E.

Green food formula and/or Vegetable Alkalizer Juice:

Take an alkalizing green formula in either a pill, powder, or liquid form and/or drink Vegetable Alkalizer Juice (see Chapter 6).

Even if you eat dark leafy greens each day, you need additional superfoods and greens to keep your body alkaline; detoxify the negative effects from radiation, chemicals, and heavy metals; and provide your body with sufficient minerals to repair itself.

Brands:
- NanoGreens[10] (BioPharma Scientific)
- Vitamineral Green (HealthForce Nutritionals)

Ground flaxseed meal:

Put one tablespoon of organic ground flaxseed meal in eight ounces of water or sprinkle on salads or vegetables. Fiber is key in keeping your bowels moving daily, sweeping debris from the colon lining, and lowering cholesterol.

Brand:
- Bob's Red Mill (keep refrigerated after opening)

Digestive enzymes (1 after each meal, optional):

Take for the second month only as needed (if you still have gas, bloating, heartburn, or constipation).

Red clover tea (work up slowly to 4 cups daily):

This herb cleanses your bloodstream, liver, and kidneys. One heaping teaspoon of the loose herb makes one cup of tea. To make four cups of the tea, bring one quart of filtered water to a boil, and turn off the heat. Add four teaspoons of the bulk herb to a large French press, add boiling water, let it steep for fifteen minutes, and then slowly push the plunger down. After brewing, you can add ice cubes to make iced tea to drink throughout the day. Make sure to consume whatever amount you make the same day or it will get moldy, even if kept in the refrigerator.

SECOND AND THIRD MONTHS: DAYS 31–90 SUPPLEMENT SCHEDULE

Supplement	Arising	Breakfast	Lunch	Dinner	Bedtime	After Meal[1]	Empty Stomach
Antifungal (dose depends on which product is used)[2]	X	Dose depends on which product is used	X (½ hour before meal)	X (½ hour before meal)			X
Vitamin C						X (pills/powder)	X (powder only)
Liver abX		1	1	1		X	
Vitamin E (400 IU)		1				X	
Ground flaxseed meal		1 tbsp any time during the day				X	
Red clover tea		4 cups daily				X	
Omega 3 fish oil		1		1		X	
Evening primrose oil (women only)		1		1		X	
Adrenal abX or Adaptocrine		1	1			X	
Green food/Veg. Alkalizer Juice				X			X
Gluco abX or Glysen (optional)		1	1	1		X	
Digestive enzymes (optional)		1	1	1		X	

1. After-meal supplements will digest better and make you feel less bloated if you take them right before your first bite of food vs. your last bite of food.

2. Antifungal: Continue taking your antifungal at the dosage where you left off at the end of the first month (may switch to a different herbal antifungal for third month). For severe cases of candida, take 2 pills 3x/day of Candida abX or Candida Cleanse.

SUPPLEMENTATION FOR ADDITIONAL NEEDS

The supplements listed below are for those who have additional and/or stubborn symptoms that need to be addressed while doing the 90-day program. Add them into the list of your daily supplementation as needed.

ELIMINATION PROBLEMS

Constipation

Herbal laxative:

Start by taking the minimum dose on the label in the evening and see if you eliminate in the morning. If you don't, increase by one pill each night after dinner until you achieve daily elimination. The goal is to have full, normal bowel movements, not diarrhea, so adjust the dose until it is right for you. If you have taken up to four pills in the evening and are still not eliminating daily then switch to another product. Magnesium citrate and triphala are milder formulas for constipation, and Aloe Lite and Aloe 225 are stronger.

Brands:
- Aloe Lite (Bio-Design)
- Aloe 225 (Bio-Design)
- Magnesium Citrate (Metagenics)
- Triphala (Planetary Herbals, Himalaya USA)

These can be used long term.

- Naturalax #2 or #3 (Nature's Way)

- Aloelax (Nature's Way)
- Dr. Christopher's Quick Colon Part 1
  (Christopher's Original Formulas)

These can be used for only six months because they have addictive stimulating herbs in them.

Aloe vera juice (4 ounces in a.m. and again in p.m. on an empty stomach):

Drink four ounces upon arising and four ounces at bedtime without food. The juice from the aloe vera plant helps reduce gastrointestinal inflammation, repair leaky gut, and alleviate constipation. The juice can be used long term.

Brands:
- Lily of the Desert
- George's Aloe Vera

Diarrhea

Psyllium seed:

This is a fiber that expands in size and helps to form normal stools.

Brand:
- Herbulk (Metagenics)

LEAKY GUT

In this condition, the lining of the GI tract is porous and irritated, causing food allergies, asthma, and weakened immunity.

It is almost a given that most people today have either mild or severe leaky gut because of our contaminated food, air, and water supply. Those with severe cases of leaky gut, indicated by such conditions as Crohn's disease, celiac disease, diverticulitis, or ulcerative colitis, or those who are taking pain medication may take one of the following formulas for an extended period of time or as needed.

RepairVite, IntestiNEW, or Glutagenics:

These herbal-vitamin powders contain the amino acid L-glutamine, aloe vera, and deglycerized licorice. They help repair leaky gut; alleviate acid reflux, heartburn, ulcers, and brain fatigue; and help stop sugar/carb cravings.

Brands:
- RepairVite, K-63, caramel flavor (Apex Energetics)
- IntestiNEW (ReNew Life)
- Glutagenics (Metagenics)

Aloe Vera juice (4 ounces in a.m. and again in p.m. on an empty stomach):

Drink four ounces upon arising and four ounces at bedtime without food. The juice from the aloe vera plant helps reduce gastrointestinal inflammation, repair leaky gut, and alleviate constipation. The juice can be used long term.

Brands:
- Lily of the Desert
- George's Aloe Vera

Endefen or Intestinal Repair Complex:

These powdered herbal-vitamin formulas support the healing of an inflamed gastric lining and promote the growth of beneficial bacteria. They are good remedies for Crohn's disease, IBS, and ulcerative colitis.

   Brand:
   - Endefen (Metagenics)
   - Intestinal Repair Complex (BioGenesis)

THYROID SUPPORT

The largest endocrine gland in the body, the thyroid sits in the neck. It is primarily responsible for how quickly the body burns energy and for regulating metabolism. Signs of low thyroid (hypothyroidism) are depression, weight gain, hair loss, puffy eyes and face, constipation, skin problems, headaches, poor circulation, fatigue, or loss of the outer third of the eyebrows. Before addressing a thyroid imbalance, it is critical to address weak adrenal function and candida overgrowth as I have described throughout the book.

Eating seaweed is the best first step to balancing your thyroid and can be started at the outset of your 90-day program. Seaweed is an excellent food source of iodine as well as minerals that can help optimize thyroid function and offset the negative effects of radiation and heavy metals. Iodine is needed by the thyroid to make thyroxine. If it cannot be produced, thyroid function will be decreased, resulting in hypothyroidism. The typical Western diet is now deficient in iodine because of depleted soils, poor diets, and a decrease in salt usage. Tri-Kelp is a good source of three seaweeds and can be added to smoothies or sprinkled on salads or other foods, using ¼ to 1 teaspoon daily (see Resources).

If thyroid balance is not achieved, consider replacing seaweed with (or adding) Thyroid abX or GTA supplements, or asking your doctor for a prescription for Armour or Nature-Throid. When using any thyroid supplements or medication, make sure to have a blood test done every three to six months in order to monitor your thyroid markers.

Thyroid formulas:

These herbal-vitamin supplements are designed to balance thyroid function and are particularly beneficial for those with autoimmune thyroid conditions, such as Hashimoto's disease. These formulas can be used long term if needed.

Brands:
- Thyroid abX (Quintessential Healing, Inc.)
- GTA or GTA Forte (Biotics Research)

Notes:
- Do not take any thyroid supplements if you are currently taking pharmaceutical thyroid medication.
- If you notice signs of hyperthyroid while taking one of these supplements (sudden weight loss, insomnia, restlessness, rapid heartbeat, sweating, increased appetite, goiter), stop taking or reduce the dosage. Have your doctor check your thyroid markers by doing blood work.

WEIGHT-GAIN REMEDIES

If you are having trouble keeping weight on, here are some suggestions. With each meal, eat a small amount of gluten-free grains (specifically brown rice) from the "Foods to Eat" list. Eat more winter squashes, such as pumpkin, butternut, acorn, etc. Eat avocado and nuts and nut butters daily. Make a protein smoothie with the protein powder listed below, using unsweetened almond, coconut, or hemp milk. Add one tablespoon of raw coconut oil (melted) or one tablespoon of almond or macadamia nut butter, and banana (allowed during the first three months for those who need to gain weight).

Whey powders:

These high-grade whey powders are made from contented cows. They are grass-fed and never subjected to growth hormone treatment, chemicals, pesticides, or genetically modified organisms (GMOs). One formula has colostrum for extra immune support. These products are allowed for the purpose of weight gain. Those sensitive to dairy might not tolerate them well.

Brands:
- NanoProPRP Immune (BioPharma Scientific)
- The True Whey (Source Naturals)

CHAPTER 8

I FEEL GREAT—
HOW DO I MAINTAIN?

O nce you're well, candida overgrowth can come back even more virulently if you go back to old habits of eating poorly. It is important for those of you with stubborn, chronic conditions, such as autoimmune diseases or cancer, to take at least a reduced dose of an herbal antifungal compound every day for the rest of your life. You will also need to increase your dosage during stressful periods, such as when traveling and during holidays.

For those of you who are not challenged with these conditions but feel that unhealthy lifestyle habits and high stress might creep back in, it's a good idea to take ongoing maintenance doses of Candida abX (one pill two times a day), pau d'arco (one cup of tea or one dropperful of tincture twice daily), or Candida Cleanse (one pill two times a day). Rotate these products every couple of months to make sure you don't become immune to any one of them. For those who are able to maintain a healthy diet, I suggest replacing your antifungal with a probiotic and taking that for the rest of your life to keep your digestive system and yeast levels in balance. Specifics about probiotics are discussed later in this chapter.

Even after you reach the end of the 90-day program, you need to be moderate with your diet. Avoid indulging in foods that contain sugar, dairy, yeast, corn, gluten, soy, and refined carbohydrates, and avoid drinking alcohol. You can keep your diet clean by eating the foods on the "Foods to Eat to Maintain Health" list at least 80 percent of the time and eating the foods on the "Foods to Eat Infrequently or Not at All" list only 20 percent of the time or less. One way to achieve this is to stick to the lists and eat healthily from Mondays through Fridays and then enjoy a little of the "no-no" foods on the weekends.

You will now be adding foods back into your diet that you haven't eaten during the 90-day protocol. If you notice intolerances and reactions after eating these foods, such as a rapid pulse (90 to 180 beats per minute), fatigue, itching internally or externally, hives, gas, bloating, headaches, or other symptoms, eliminate those foods. This is a clear sign your body does not want them in your system.

Continue to drink red clover tea each week, as it clears environmental toxins and removes stress hormones from the bloodstream. Stop drinking it for a month three times a year so that you don't become allergic to it, or switch to dandelion root tea during that month. You can reduce your intake of red clover to two cups three or four times a week, and drink four cups when you are under stress and/or your diet is poor.

Digestive enzymes are good to take during times of travel, high stress, eating poorly, and going to bed on a full stomach.

FOODS TO EAT TO
MAINTAIN HEALTH
(EAT AT LEAST 80% OF THE TIME)

Animal Protein (antibiotic- and hormone-free as much as possible)

Beef, buffalo, lamb (grass-fed; once a week; eat with greens and not
   with starchy vegetables, beans, or grains)
Chicken, duck, and turkey
Eggs (organic or pasture-raised, if possible)
Fish (limit shellfish to once or twice a month)

Note: Due to ongoing ocean pollution from many sources, including
   nuclear leaks at the Fukushima Daiichi power plant in Japan, stay up
   to date on which fish become contaminated.

Grains (whole and unrefined only)

Amaranth
Breads (gluten-, sugar-, dairy-, yeast-free)
Brown, black, or wild rice (limit to 2–3 times a week)
Buckwheat
Crackers (brown rice and flax; limit to 2–3 times a week)
Kañiwa
Millet
Oats (gluten-free)
Pasta (gluten- and corn-free; limit to once a week)
Quinoa
Sorghum
Tapioca
Teff
Yucca

Oils (cold-pressed only)

Almond oil (can be used for cooking)
Avocado oil (can be used for cooking
Coconut oil (can be used for cooking)
Flaxseed oil (not for cooking)
Grapeseed oil (can be used for cooking)

Hempseed oil (not for cooking)
Olive oil (can be used for cooking)
Pistachio oil (not for cooking)
Safflower oil (can be used for cooking)
Red Palm Fruit oil (can be used for cooking, low heat only)
Sesame oil (can be used for cooking)
Sunflower-seed oil (can be used for cooking)
Walnut oil (not for cooking)

Note: At restaurants, eat what is served; be more stringent when using oils at home

Nuts and Seeds (raw; unroasted if commercial; may dry-roast your own)

Almonds
Brazil
Cashews
Chestnuts
Chia seeds
Flaxseeds
Hazelnuts
Hempseeds
Macadamia
Nut butters (all except peanut butter; nut butters can be dry-roasted)
Pecans
Pine nuts
Pistachios
Pumpkin seeds and pumpkin-seed butter
Sesame seeds (also raw tahini butter)
Sunflower seeds and sunflower-seed butter
Walnuts

Note: Limit quantity to a small handful at a time, and chew thoroughly.

Dairy (antibiotic- and hormone-free only)

Butter (small amounts, unsalted; preferably organic from grass-fed cows)
Clarified butter (ghee, organic)
Goat and sheep cheeses (raw,* once or twice a month)

Vegetables (60% of your daily diet; dark-green leafy vegetables and cruciferous vegetables are most important)

All (except mushrooms, potatoes, and corn)

*Pregnant and nursing women should not eat raw dairy products.

Condiments

Apple cider vinegar (raw, unfiltered only—store in refrigerator)

Bragg Liquid Aminos (unfermented soy sauce; only acceptable soy product)

Dill relish (made without vinegar; Bubbies)

Dry mustard (or small amounts of mustard made with apple cider vinegar)

Fresh herbs (basil, parsley, etc.)

Mayonnaise (small amounts made with safflower oil, or use home-made in Recipes section)

Pepper

Rice vinegar (unseasoned and unsweetened only—store in the refrigerator)

Sea salt

Spices (without sugar, MSG, or additives; favor ginger and turmeric, which are anti-inflammatory)

Beverages

Bragg Apple Cider Vinegar Drinks (Ginger Spice, Limeade, and Sweet Stevia only)

Fresh coconut water (only during or right after exercise, 14 grams of sugar in a can)

Green tea (caffeinated or decaffeinated)

Herbal teas (red clover, peppermint, etc.)

Suja Water (Lemon Love)

Unsweetened almond, coconut, or hemp milk

Unsweetened mineral water (Gerolsteiner, Perrier)

Water (filtered, purified, or distilled only)

Beans and Legumes

All (organic, small amounts; but no soybeans, tofu, or tempeh)

Miscellaneous

Cacao powder (raw, unsweetened)

Carob (unsweetened)

Cocoa powder (unsweetened)

Coconut butter (organic)

Dill pickles (made without vinegar only; Bubbies)

Gums/mints (sweetened with lo han, stevia, or xylitol)

Salsa (without sugar or vinegar, except apple cider vinegar)

Sauerkraut (made without vinegar only; Bubbies)

Fruits (1–2 fruits a day)

All berries
All citrus fruits
All dried fruits (apricots, dates, figs, raisins, cranberries, prunes; limit
   to 1–2 times per month, high in sugar)
All melons
Apples
Apricots
Avocado*
Bananas
Cherries
Coconut (small amounts of coconut water, high in sugar)
Grapes (small amounts, high in sugar)
Lemons, limes*
Kiwis
Mangoes
Nectarines
Papayas
Peaches
Pears
Persimmon
Pineapples
Plums
Pomegranates

Sweeteners

Chicory root (Just Like Sugar)
Lo han (luo han, monk fruit extract)
Stevia
Xylitol (small amounts; The Ultimate Sweetener, Xyla)

*Avocado and lemon or lime juice can be in addition to your 1–2 fruits
   per day.

FOODS TO EAT INFREQUENTLY OR NOT AT ALL

(EAT 20% OF THE TIME OR LESS)

Animal Protein

Bacon (except turkey bacon without nitrates and hormones; gluten-free)

Hotdogs (except chicken or turkey hotdogs without nitrates and hormones; gluten-free; small amounts because high in sodium)

Processed and packaged meats

Sausages (except chicken and turkey without added sugar, hormones, and nitrates; gluten-free)

Shellfish, farmed fish, GMO salmon, tuna (all: toro, albacore, ahi, etc., including canned)

Oils

Canola oil (small amounts okay)

Corn oil

Cottonseed oil

Partially hydrogenated or hydrogenated oils

Peanut oil

Soy oil

Vegetables

Corn

Mushrooms

Potatoes

Nuts and Seeds

Peanuts, peanut butter

Dairy

Cheeses (all, including cottage and cream cheese)

Buttermilk

Cow's milk

Goat's milk

Ice cream

Margarine

Sour cream
Yogurt (unless plain in raw dairy base and antibiotic- and hormone-
free)

Grains

Barley
Breads (refined)
Cereals (dry, except gluten- and sugar-free)
Corn
Crackers (white flour, gluten)
Farro
Kamut
Pasta (except corn- and gluten-free)
Pastries
Popcorn
Rye
Spelt
Triticale
White rice
White flours
Wheat (refined and whole)

Condiments

Gravy
Jams and jellies
Ketchup
Mayonnaise (except small amounts with safflower oil or homemade in
Recipes section)
Pickles
Relish
Salad dressing (unless sugar-free and made with apple cider vinegar or
unsweetened rice vinegar)
Sauces with vinegars and sugar
Soy sauce, ponzu, and tamari sauce
Spices that contain yeast, sugar, or additives, such as MSG

Beans and Legumes

Soybeans (tofu, tempeh)

Miscellaneous

Candy
Chocolate (dark, if you do indulge)
Cookies
Donuts
Fast food and fried foods
Fruit strips
Gelatin

Gum (unless sweetened with lo han, stevia, or xylitol)
Jerky (beef, turkey)
Lozenges/mints (unless sweetened with lo han, stevia, or xylitol)
Muffins
Pastries
Pizza
Popcorn
Processed food (TV dinners, etc.)
Smoked, dried, pickled, and cured foods

Beverages

Alcohol
Coffee, including decaffeinated (if you do indulge, drink espresso,
   organic only, 1 cup per day maximum)
Energy drinks (e.g., Red Bull, Gatorade, etc.)
Fruit juices
Kefir (pasteurized)
Kombucha
Rice milk
Sodas (diet and regular)
Soy milk

Fruits

All juices (sweetened or unsweetened)
All dried fruits (apricots, dates, figs, raisins, sweetened cranberries,
   prunes, etc.)

Sweeteners

Agave nectar/syrup (Nectevia)
Artificial sweeteners, such as aspartame (Nutrasweet), acesulfame K,
   saccharin, and sucralose (Splenda)
Barley malt
Brown rice syrup
Brown sugar
Coconut nectar/sugar
Corn syrup, dextrose, maltodextrin
Erythritol (Nectresse, Swerve, Truvia)
Fructose, products sweetened with fruit juice
Honey (raw and processed)
Maltitol
Mannitol
Maple syrup
Molasses
Raw or evaporated cane juice crystals
Sorbitol
White sugar
Yacon syrup

WHAT IF I NEED TO TAKE AN ANTIBIOTIC?

There are those critical times when you may need to take an antibiotic for a bacterial infection such as pneumonia, staph, strep, or Helicobacter pylori. If your doctor prescribes an antibiotic and you choose to take it, ask for Diflucan (fluconazole), three tablets total, to take after you finish the antibiotic. Take probiotics (Flora 20-14, 11-Strain Probiotic Powder, or Ultimate Flora) while on the antibiotic, but at a different time of the day. After your antibiotic course, take one Diflucan tablet every three days. Take the probiotics while you're taking the Diflucan, but at a different time, and continue the probiotics for one more month. Then switch to two months of herbal antifungals such as Candida abX or Candida Cleanse.

Doctors usually don't offer antifungals, but they need to be willing to give them to you if you ask. If your doctor won't give you three tablets, then just get one pill, as that is better than nothing. If you can't get Diflucan, take one month of probiotics and then switch to taking the antifungal you have been taking while on the program (e.g., Candida abX, Candida Cleanse, or Nystatin).

If you are not ambulatory, but have started the antifungal and supplement protocol and are feeling stronger and eliminating daily, you should be able to handle Diflucan. However, if you are weak and fragile or haven't started the program yet, use only the probiotics.

SUPPLEMENTATION FOR QUALITY AGING

To keep yourself balanced and to experience quality aging, follow the recommendations below after you finish your 90-day program.

FOURTH MONTH AND ONGOING

New Food Lists to Use as a Guide

- Eat foods from the "Foods to Eat to Maintain Health" list (see page 175). Slowly introduce any new foods back into your diet. If you have a bad reaction, this is your body's way of telling you to stay away from that food or to indulge in it less frequently.
- Avoid the foods on the "Foods to Eat Infrequently or Not at All" list or eat them only 20 percent of the time or less (see page 179).

Supplements to Take

Probiotics (dairy-free strains of acidophilus and bifidus):

Probiotics replace and balance bacteria in the GI tract. Take as directed on the bottle, typically twice a day on an empty stomach. If you are disciplined by nature and can maintain a healthy diet and minimal stress, taking the probiotic for the rest of your life should be sufficient to keep you free from candida overgrowth. However, for most people, stress and poor diet more often prevail. In these cases, to stay balanced it is best to take a probiotic as well as an herbal antifungal for the rest of your life, as described below.

Brands:
- Flora 20-14 (Innate Response, refrigerate)
- 11-Strain Probiotic Powder (Custom Probiotics, refrigerate)
- Ultimate Flora RTS 15 billion (ReNew Life, no refrigeration required)
- Primal Defense Ultra (Garden of Life, no refrigeration required)

Herbal antifungal (only for those who have continual high stress and do not maintain a clean diet):

As stated above, taking a probiotic for the rest your life (without an antifungal) is sufficient if you can maintain a clean diet and low stress levels. Those who find it too challenging to do this would do best to take a probiotic as well as an antifungal in order to stay balanced. To make sure that you don't become immune to a particular antifungal formula, remember to rotate the different formulas every couple of months, as described on page 173 (Candida abX, pau d'arco tea or tincture, and Candida Cleanse). Take the antifungal for one or two months, and then take probiotics for a month. Continue this cycle for life. Alternatively, you can take both antifungals and probiotics in the same month, but at different times of the day. Take your antifungal with meals, and take only one pill (instead of two) of your probiotic per day, either before sleep or between meals on an empty stomach.

Multivitamin-mineral supplement:

A good multivitamin-mineral supplement will compensate for some of the nutrients that are missing in your diet. Make sure your source has chelated minerals (minerals bound with amino acids to improve digestion) and no iron. If you are anemic and need additional iron, use food-based brands; synthetic iron can be toxic to the brain. Iron Response by Innate Response and HemeVite by Apex Energetics are good sources and are non-constipating.

Brands:
- Life Force Multiple No Iron capsules (Source Naturals)
- Two-Per-Day Capsules (Life Extension)

B-complex vitamins (optional):

If you are taking a one-a-day multivitamin-mineral supplement as opposed to a brand that you are supposed to take twice or three times a day, you will need to take an extra B-complex supplement. B-complex vitamins are a must for vegetarians because certain B vitamins are lacking in a vegetarian diet.

Brands:
- Glucogenics (Metagenics)
- B-Right (Jarrow Formulas)

Vitamin C (300–700 mg whole food source or 2,000 mg daily):

Buy a vitamin C that contains a whole-food source or one with mineral ascorbates and/or bioflavonoids. Plain ascorbic acid crystals will irritate the lining of your stomach and intestines. Spread out the dosage through the day because your body will absorb only so much at one time. Increase your dose of vitamin C slowly. If you experience diarrhea, cut back your dose. You can take powders with or without food, but it's best to take pills after a meal or snack. A multivitamin-mineral does contain vitamin C, but does not have high enough amounts for quality aging.

Brands:
- Truly Natural Vitamin C powder (HealthForce Nutritionals)
- QBC Plex (Solaray)
- Super-C Plus, tablets or powder (Dr. Schulze's)

Vitamin E (400 IU daily):

When buying vitamin E, be sure the source is natural. Look for "d-tocopherol" on the label and not "dl-tocopherol," which is synthetic. Also use an E vitamin that has mixed tocopherols and tocotrienols. A multivitamin-mineral does contain vitamin E, but does not have high enough amounts for quality aging.

Brands:
- E Gems Elite (Carlson)
- familE (Jarrow Formulas)

Notes:
- Do not take vitamin E if you are on blood thinners.
- If you will be having surgery, stop taking vitamin E two weeks prior so your blood will clot properly.
- If you begin to bruise easily, reduce your dosage of vitamin E.

Green food formula and/or Vegetable Alkalizer Juice:

Take an alkalizing green formula in either a pill, powder, or liquid form and/or drink Vegetable Alkalizer Juice (see Chapter 6). Even if you eat dark leafy greens each day, you need additional superfoods and greens to keep your body alkaline; to detoxify the negative effects from radiation, chemicals, and heavy metals; and to provide your body with sufficient minerals to repair itself.

Brands:
- NanoGreens[10] (BioPharma Scientific)
- Vitamineral Green (HealthForce Nutritionals)

Free-form amino acid complex (2 pills upon arising; if it irritates your stomach, take after breakfast):

Amino acids are the building blocks of protein that are responsible for repairing and regenerating every cell, tissue, and organ in your body. They also assist the liver's detoxification process and are the precursors to neurotransmitters such as serotonin, dopamine, and epinephrine.

Brands:
- AminoBlend (Douglas Labs 740 mg)
- Max-Amino Caps (Country Life)

Omega-3 fish oil (1,200–1,500 mg daily with food):

This essential fatty acid is not manufactured by the body. It helps decrease inflammation, feed brain and nerve cells, and support cardiovascular function. It is important to buy a brand that is free of PCBs (carcinogenic, manmade chemicals used in electrical equipment and industrial processes). The brands I have listed below are PCB-free.

Brands:
- OmegaGenics EPA-DHA 720 (Metagenics)
- Ultimate Omega-3 fish oil gels (Nordic Naturals)
- Elite Omega-3 Gems Fish Oil, Professional Strength (Carlson)

Note:
- Do not take fish oil if you are on blood-thinning medication. If you will be having surgery, stop taking the fish oil two weeks before so your blood will clot properly.

Evening primrose oil (1,000 mg daily: 500 mg twice a day—for women only):

This is an omega-6 essential fatty acid that is rich in gamma linoleic acid (GLA), which assists in balancing female hormones and eliminating PMS symptoms.

Brands:
- Evening Primrose Oil (Jarrow Formulas, NOW Foods)

Vitamin D3 (2,000 IU):

Vitamin D is a fat-soluble vitamin that has many functions, from contributing to bone health to supporting immune function. Even though the body manufactures vitamin D when skin is exposed to ultraviolet radiation from the sun, most people today are found to have low levels. Vitamin D3 (cholecalciferol) is the best supplement form to take. You can easily have your blood tested to see if your vitamin D levels are out of range and how much you need. Those with autoimmune diseases would take higher amounts of 4,000–8,000 IU daily to ensure that their blood levels are in the range of 60–80 ng/mL.

Brands:
- Vitamin D3 (Jarrow)
- Vitamin D3 (Life Extension)
- Vitamin D3 (D-Mulsion liquid drops; Biotics Research)

Ground flaxseed meal:

Put one tablespoon of organic ground flaxseed meal in eight ounces of water or sprinkle on salads or vegetables. Fiber is key in keeping your bowels moving daily, sweeping debris from the colon lining, and lowering cholesterol.

Brand:
- Bob's Red Mill

FOURTH MONTH AND ONGOING SUPPLEMENT SCHEDULE

Supplement	Arising	Breakfast	Lunch	Dinner	Bedtime	After Meal[1]	Empty Stomach
Probiotics or Antifungal[2]	X				X		X
Vitamin C		Dose depends on which product used				X (pills/powder)	X (powder only)
Multivitamin-mineral		Dose depends on which product used				X	
Amino acid complex	2						X
Vitamin E (400 IU)		1				X	
Vitamin D3 (2,000 IU)		X				X	
Green food/Veg. Alkalizer Juice			X				X
Ground flaxseed meal		1 tbsp any time during the day				X	X
Omega 3 fish oil		1		1		X	
Evening Primrose Oil (women only)		1		1		X	
Red clover tea[3]		2–4 cups, 3 or 4 times a week				X	X
Digestive enzyme (optional)		1	1	1		X	
B-complex (optional)			1			X	

1. After-meal supplements will digest better and make you feel less bloated if you take them right before your first bite of food vs. your last bite of food.

2. Probiotics: 11-Strain Probiotic Powder, Flora 20-14, Ultimate Flora RTS 15 billion, or Primal Defense Ultra (amount indicated on bottle when arising and at bedtime). If you will be alternating probiotics with antifungals on different months as explained on page 184, when using the antifungal, take 1 pill 3 times a day ½ hour before a meal, or after meals if it upsets your stomach. Check probiotics label to see if refrigeration is required.

3. Continue to drink red clover tea each week, but stop drinking it for a month 3 times a year so you don't become allergic to it, or switch to dandelion root tea during that month.

RECAPTURING YOUR VITALITY

You now have everything you need to begin your journey of redefining your lifestyle habits so that you can feel vibrantly healthy again. This program will help you to look and feel your best and give you the energy and motivation necessary to fulfill your goals and dreams. Just remember that your body cannot take care of itself. You need to keep up the required maintenance, just as when you regularly change the oil in your car to keep it running smoothly.

The secret is to keep your mind-set away from deprivation and focus on the primary purpose of this program—to remove infection and inflammation from your body so you can recapture your energy, clarity, and vitality. Ninety days is a very short period of time in which to do this. As you progress, you will enjoy hearing the comments from your family, friends, and colleagues about how great you look. Though this may be gratifying, the best part is that you will feel great inside too!

NOTES

CHAPTER 1

1. Michael J. Goldberg, "Autism and the Immune Connection," http://www.neuroimmunedr.com/articles.html.
2. Christina M. Hull, Ryan M. Raisner, and Alexander D. Johnson, "Evidence for Mating of the 'Asexual' Yeast *Candida albicans* in a Mammalian Host," *Science* 289, no. 5477 (July 2000).
3. C. Orian Truss, *The Missing Diagnosis* (Birmingham, AL: The Missing Diagnosis, Inc., 1985), 24.
4. Michael J. Kennedy and Paul A. Volz, "Ecology of *Candida albicans* Gut Colonization: Inhibition of Candida Adhesion, Colonization, and Dissemination from the Gastrointestinal Tract by Bacterial Antagonism," *Infection and Immunity*, September 1985, 49(3): 654–63, quoted in John P. Trowbridge and Morton Walker, *The Yeast Syndrome: How to Help Your Doctor Identify and Treat the Real Cause of Your Yeast-Related Illness* (New York: Bantam Books, 1986), 49.
5. Ibid, 9.
6. J. P. Nolan, "Intestinal Endotoxins as Mediators of Hepatic Injury— an Idea Whose Time Has Come Again," *Hepatology* 10, no. 5 (November 1989): 887–91.
7. C. Orian Truss, *The Missing Diagnosis* (Birmingham, AL: The Missing Diagnosis, Inc., 1985), 46.

CHAPTER 2

1. M. Percival, *Functional Dietetics: The Core of Health Integration* (Ontario, Canada: Health Coach Systems International, 1995).
2. Jeffrey S. Bland, "Leaky Gut: A Common Problem with Food Allergies," interview by Marjorie Hurt Jones, RN, *Mastering Food Allergies Newsletter* VIII, no. 5 (September–October 1993).

3. N. Klotz and N. Ulrich, "Natural Benzodiazepines in Man," *Lancet* 335 (1990): 992.

CHAPTER 3

1. John P. Trowbridge and Morton Walker, *The Yeast Syndrome: How to Help Your Doctor Identify and Treat the Real Cause of Your Yeast-Related Illness* (New York: Bantam Books, 1986), 129.

CHAPTER 4

1. Ann Louise Gittleman, *How to Stay Young and Healthy in a Toxic World* (Chicago: Keats Publishing, 1999), 19.
2. Sharon Begley, "The End of Antibiotics," *Newsweek* 123, no. 13 (March 28, 1994): 48.
3. W. F. Nieuwenhuizen et al., "Is Candida Albicans a Trigger in the Onset of Coeliac Disease?" *Lancet* 361, no. 9375 (June 2003).
4. Marios Hadjivassiliou et al., "Gluten Sensitivity: From Gut to Brain," *Lancet Neurology* 9, no. 3 (March 2010): 318–30.
5. F. Batmanghelidj, *Your Body's Many Cries for Water* (Falls Church, VA: Global Health Solutions, Inc., 1995), 69.
6. F. Batmanghelidj, *Water for Health, for Healing, for Life: You're Not Sick, You're Thirsty!* (New York: Warner Books, 2003), 185.

RESOURCES

Supplements and Other Products

abX Products from Quintessential Healing, Inc.

www.annboroch.com (Products page)

Products: Adaptocrine, Adrenal abX, Candida abX, Gallbladder abX, Gluco abX, Glysen, HemeVite, Liver abX, RepairVite (K-63, caramel flavor), Thyroid abX

Bio-Design

(800) 822-6193 (say you were referred by Ann Boroch)

Products: Aloe Lite, Aloe 225

Custom Probiotics

www.customprobiotics.com

Product: 11-Strain Probiotic Powder

Dr. Schulze's Original Clinical Formulae

www.herbdoc.com

Products: Super-C Plus, Powder or Tablets

Emerson Ecologics

High-grade professional line of vitamins, supplements, and herbs

www.emersonecologics.com   (800) 654-4432

Tell customer service that you want to set up a patient account under Ann Boroch and give the code Quint1 and 91604.

Brands: BioPharma Scientific, Douglas Laboratories, Innate Response, Priority One

General Ecology, Inc.

www.generalecology.com/products.php   (800) 441-8166

Products: Water filtration systems, including portable system using structured matrix technology

Ionic Researchers Association

www.annboroch.com (click on Products page)

Product: Ionic S.P.A. (footbath)

Long Life Unlimited

www.longlifeunlimited.com/category.sc?categoryId=69

(877) 433-3962

Product: Aclare Air purifier

Mendocino Medicinal

www.mendocinomedicinal.com   (707) 459-2101

Products: Tri-Kelp (sea cabbage, bull kelp, palm kelp)—source of iodine to help maintain healthy thyroid function and to offset negative effects of radiation and heavy-metal buildup in the body. Consume ¼ to 1 teaspoon daily in a smoothie or with food. Company also supplies topical compounds for pain and skin afflictions.

Mountain Rose Herbs

www.mountainroseherbs.com

(800) 879-3337

Products: Organic bulk herbs: dandelion root, hibiscus, red clover dried herb, pau d'arco, chamomile, peppermint

Vitamin Warehouses

These online warehouses sell vitamins, food, and natural body-care products at reduced prices.

www.vitacost.com

www.amazon.com

www.iherb.com

Brands: Bio-Design, BioPharma Scientific, Biotics Research, Bob's Red Mill, Carlson, Christopher's, Douglas Laboratories, Essential Formulas, Enzymedica, Gaia Herbs, Garden of Life, George's, HealthForce Nutritionals, Himalaya USA, Jarrow Formulas, Life Extension, Lily of the Desert, Made in U.S.A., Metagenics, Nature's Way, Nordic Naturals, NOW Foods, Planetary Herbals, Priority One, Rainbow Light, ReNew Life, Solaray, Source Naturals

Manufacturers and Suppliers
of Specialty Foods and Beverages

The majority of products I recommend can be ordered on amazon.com, vitacost.com, and iherb.com, or by going directly to the manufacturers' websites, including those listed below, if you cannot find them in your local health food store.

Alchemy Foods

www.alchemyfoods.net

Products: Candidly Cookies and Candidly Granola

Awesome Foods

www.awesomefoods.com

Products: Raw breads and chips

Basiltops

www.basiltops.com

Products: Dairy-free spicy and non-spicy pestos

Bragg

www.bragg.com

Products: Unfermented, non-GMO soy sauce; kelp seasoning; and stevia-sweetened beverages

Coconut Secret

www.coconutsecret.com

Products: Raw Coconut Aminos, Raw Coconut Flour

DNA Life Bars

www.dnalifebars.com

Enter coupon code borochio to save 10% or go to www.anboroch .com and order from the Products page.

Products: Protein squares and treats

Food for Life

www.foodforlife.com

Products: Brown Rice Tortillas, Black Rice Tortillas

Go Raw

www.goraw.com

Products: Cereals, chips, crackers, nuts, and seeds

Jilz Snackerz

www.jilzsnackerz.com

Products: Jilz Gluten Free Crackerz

Just Poppin

www.justpoppin.com

Products: Tru-Pop Popping Sorghum

Lydia's Organics

www.lydiasorganics.com

Products: Raw breads, cereals, chips, and crackers

Majestic Garlic

www.majesticgarlic.com/index.php

Products: Garlic spreads in various flavors

Mauk Family Farms

www.maukfamilyfarms.com

Products: Flax crackers and crusts

Nut Just a Cookie

www.nutjustacookie.com

Products: Nutty Nibbles cookies; choose sugar-free varieties

Rox Chox

www.roxchox.blogspot.com/p/all-about-rox-chox.html

Products: Organic chocolate treats sweetened with xylitol; made with raw cacao and coconut

Sami's Bakery

www.samisbakery.com

Products: Millet & Flax Bread, Lavash (Wait at least 90 days to integrate any of their other millet and flax products because of added sugars; and even then, eat only small amounts, as they may aggravate candida in some people's bodies and cause bloating.

Sea Tangle Noodle Company

www.kelpnoodles.com/index.html

Products: Kelp noodles

Steve's PaleoGoods

www.stevespaleogoods.com

Product: Steve's Original Paleo Stix (grass-fed beef sticks)

Two Moms in the Raw

www.twomomsintheraw.com

Products: Flax crackers

Books on Candida

Boroch, Ann. *The Candida Cure*. Quintessential Healing Publishing, Inc., 2012.

Crook, William G., MD. *The Yeast Connection: A Medical Breakthrough*. Vintage Books, 1986.

_____. *The Yeast Connection Handbook*. Square One Publishers, 2007.

_____. *Yeast Connection Success Stories: A Collection of Stories from People Who Are Winning the Battle Against Devastating Illness*. Square One Publishers, 2007.

Crook, William G., MD, with Elizabeth B. Crook and Hyla Cass. *The Yeast Connection and Women's Health*. Square One Publishers, 2007.

Kaufmann, Doug A. *The Fungus Link to Health Problems*. MediaTrition, 2010.

Perlmutter, David, MD. *BrainRecovery.com: Powerful Therapy for Challenging Brain Disorders*. Perlmutter Health Center, 2000.

_____. Grain Brain: *The Surprising Truth about Wheat, Carbs, and Sugar—Your Brain's Silent Killers*. Little, Brown and Company, 2013.

Perlmutter, David, MD, and Alberto Villoldo, PhD. *Power Up Your Brain*. Hay House, 2012.

Trowbridge, John P., MD, and Morton Walker, DPM. *The Yeast Syndrome: How to Help Your Doctor Identify and Treat the Real Cause of Your Yeast-Related Illness*. Bantam Books, 1986.

Truss, C. Orian, MD, *The Missing Diagnosis*. Missing Diagnosis, Inc., 1985.

Truss, C. Orian, MD, *The Missing Diagnosis II*. Missing Diagnosis, Inc., 2009.

Cookbooks

NOTE: Follow your "Foods to Eat" list, as there are differences in what some candida and allergy books allow and don't allow. You can also do an Internet search by typing in "candida recipes" and find many free recipes. Make sure to alter ingredients to match your "Foods to Eat" list.

Boroch, Ann, CNC. *The Candida Cure Cookbook*. Quintessential Healing, Inc., 2015.

Connolly, Pat, and Associates of the Price-Pottenger Nutrition Foundation. *The Candida Albicans Yeast-Free Cookbook: How Good Nutrition Can Help Fight the Epidemic of Yeast-Related Diseases*. McGraw-Hill, 2nd edition, 2000. Crook, William G., MD, and Marge H. Jones, RN. *The Yeast Connection Cookbook: A Guide to Good Nutrition and Better Health*. Square One Publishers, 2007.

Greenberg, Ronald, MD, and Angela Nori. *Freedom from Allergy Cookbook*. Blue Poppy Press, 2000.

Jones, Marjorie H., RN. *The Allergy Self-Help Cookbook*. Rodale Books, 2001.

Martin, Jeanne Marie, and Zoltan P. Rona. *Complete Candida Yeast Guidebook: Everything You Need to Know About Prevention, Treatment & Diet*, rev. 2nd ed. Prima Health, 2000.

Turner, Kristina. *The Self-Healing Cookbook: Whole Foods to Balance Body, Mind and Moods*. Earthtones Press, rev. ed., 2002.

Magazines on Nutrition and Health

Life Extension (monthly magazine, also a supplement company) www.lifeextensionretail.com

Townsend Letter (monthly magazine)

www.townsendletter.com

(360) 385-6021

Well Being Journal (magazine published 6 times a year)

www.wellbeingjournal.com

(775) 887-1702

Natural Health and Advocacy Websites

These natural health newsletters and websites provide information on nutrition, supplements, advocacy, and natural solutions for healing.

www.anh-usa.org (Alliance for Natural Health)

www.livestrong.com

www.mercola.com

www.naturalcures.com

www.naturalnews.com

www.thenhf.com (The National Health Federation)

www.organicconsumers.org (Organic Consumers Association)

www.price-pottenger.org (Price-Pottenger Nutrition Foundation)

Books and Resources on Mind-Body Healing

Byrne, Rhonda. *The Secret* (DVD): a film that can help you change your life for the better. Prime Time Productions, 2006. See http://www .thesecret.tv/index.html.

Chopra, Deepak. *Quantum Healing: Exploring the Frontiers of Mind/Body Medicine*. Bantam, 1990.

Dawson, Jasmine Contor. *Aliens to Zebras*. Tao Song, 2005.

Dwoskin, Hale. *The Sedona Method: Your Key to Lasting Happiness, Success, Peace and Emotional Well-Being*. Sedona Press, 2003.

Emotional Freedom Technique, http://www.emofree.com. This therapeutic technique helps you to release fears, phobias, addictions, cravings, and fear-based and negative thoughts and emotions.

Hay, Louise L. *You Can Heal Your Life.* Hay House, 1999.

I Can Be Fearless app.

Kasl, Charlotte. *If the Buddha Got Stuck: A Handbook for Change on a Spiritual Path.* Penguin Books, 2005.

Lipton, Bruce H. *The Biology of Belief: Unleashing the Power of Consciousness, Matter, & Miracles.* Hay House, 2008.

Maté, Gabor, MD. *When the Body Says No: Exploring the Stress-Disease Connection.* Wiley, 2011.

Myss, Caroline, PhD. *Anatomy of the Spirit.* Three Rivers Press, 1997.

Pert, Candace B. *Molecules of Emotion: The Science Behind Mind-Body Medicine.* Touchstone, 1997.

Siegel, Bernie S. *Love, Medicine and Miracles.* Random House, 1999.

Sincero, Jen. *You Are a Badass: How to Stop Doubting Your Greatness and Start Living an Awesome Life.* Running Press, 2013.

Spadaro, Patricia. *Honor Yourself: The Inner Art of Giving and Receiving.* Three Wings Press, 2009.

Tolle, Eckhart. *The Power of Now: A Guide to Spiritual Enlightenment.* New World Library, 2004.

Wilde, Stuart. *Infinite Self: 33 Steps to Reclaiming Your Inner Power.* Hay House, 1996.

Health Documentaries

Bought (2014)
The Business of Disease (2014)
Doctored (2012)
Food, Inc. (2008)
Fat, Sick & Nearly Dead (2010)
Fast Food Nation (2006)
Food Matters (2008)
Fresh (2009)
The Future of Food (2004)
Genetic Roulette: The Gamble of Our Lives (2012)

Hungry for Change (2013)

King Corn: You Are What You Eat (2007)

A Delicate Balance: The Truth (2008)

Processed People (2009)

Unacceptable Levels (2012)

Laboratories

Diagnos-Techs

Salivary hormonal testing

www.diagnostechs.com

(206) 251-0596

Cyrex Laboratories

Multi-tissue antibody testing for autoimmune conditions, gluten intolerance, and cross-reactivity food sensitivities

www.cyrexlabs.com

(602) 759-1245

Direct Labs

www.directlabs.com

(800) 908-0000

Lab provides blood chemistry panels without needing a doctor's prescription, including the Apex 4 panel (a full blood chemistry panel with a vitamin D test)

Genova Diagnostics

Stool and blood testing for candida, parasites, and gluten intolerance

www.gdx.net

(800) 522-4762

Metametrix Clinical Laboratory

Metabolic, toxicant, and nutritional testing

www.metametrix.com

(800) 221-4640

ABOUT THE AUTHOR

Ann Boroch is a certified nutritional consultant, naturopath, educator, author, and inspirational speaker. She specializes in allergies, autoimmune diseases, and gastrointestinal and endocrine disorders and is an expert on candida. Her successful practice in Los Angeles, California, has helped thousands of clients achieve optimum health.

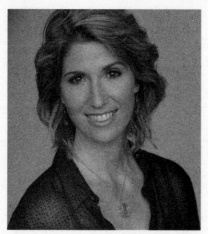

PHOTO BY OG PHOTOGRAPHY

Ann's passion is to help people realize that the body has an innate intelligence that allows it to heal itself—the key is to give it the right environment for a long enough period of time to remove inflammation and infection. She firmly believes that with choice and diligence, each of us has the power to overcome any challenge.

Ann has appeared on national radio and television, including a feature appearance on *The Montel Williams Show*, where she discussed healing multiple sclerosis.

For more information, contact:
  Website: www.annboroch.com
  Email: contact@annboroch.com
  Phone: (818) 763-8282